# TECH-PECKED OR TUNED IN:

# FINDING GOD IN A DIGITAL WORLD

# TECH-PECKED OR TUNED IN:

# FINDING GOD IN A DIGITAL WORLD

Linda Newton
and
Dr. Beverly Rodgers

ISBN: 978-1-58930-314-0
LCCN: 2019919006

# Contents

# Introduction

Do you need to...

- Understand how digital distractions generate anxiety that taxes your body and your brain and what to do about it?
- Find insights to get the best life hacks that tech provides without the vices your devices can create?
- Learn to be present in the present as you seek to connect with real live people right in front of you instead of digital substitutes?
- Experience greater productivity and creative flow as you learn how to set boundaries with multitasking?
- Discover ways to quiet your mind in a world addicted to noise and speed so that you can idle down and connect with a caring God?

Then this is the book for you.

We are identical twin sisters who love each other and love to write, so it was a delight to hear each other's ideas, share, and spend time together on this project. We are both counselors: Linda is a pastoral counselor in California with a tremendous gift for evangelism that I have always loved and admired. You will see her heart spread all over these pages. I (Beverly) am a Christian counselor who treats people with all kinds of issues in the counseling center that my husband and I run in North Carolina. I approach this subject primarily from a psychological and neurobiological perspective, dealing with the mind and brain functions as they are impacted by technology.

As Christian counselors on both the East and West Coasts, we have seen how the excessive use of technology can damage our serenity and our relationships with ourselves, others, and God. Even as I write this, I am sitting in a café near a couple eating lunch. They are technically "together" while both peruse their cell phones. At a table across from me sits a family with preteen boys. Dad has not put his phone down the entire meal. To my right are two women who have books spread in front of them and are engaging in what appears to be a book study. I have quit counting the number of selfies they have taken. And here I am on my computer, writing about the questions we all need to be asking: What is wrong with this picture? What is happening to our connections with real people?

In our counseling practices, we treat countless individuals who believe that they need to stay connected to their digital devices, yet all the while their true connections are crumbling around them. With the World Wide Web at our fingertips, people can feel greatly empowered, but current research warns of the pitfalls of too much tech time. Living with the constant bombardment from digital interruptions, we want to help people build a case for the benefit of balancing tech connections and winding down to find true connections with others right in front of us and God.

You will read extensive research on tech usage. As you will see, not balancing the time we spend on our tech devices can lead to what we call being tech-pecked. This is a term we have coined to describe the detrimental conditions that arise from the vigilant response of tech users to every ping, ding, or buzz, real or imagined, a result of a constant dependence on digital devices.

We offer a non-extreme approach to combat tech-pecked alert overload that utilizes practical protocols, sound counseling tools, and biblical insights. These are supported by real-life stories of people who have learned to idle down and balance their use of technology on all levels. This has enabled them in turn to become tuned in to a viable and thriving relationship with those close to them and with a caring God. While their names have been changed to protect their anonymity, we are grateful and honored to share their stories of victory and health. They stand as inspiring examples of people who moved from being Tech-Pecked to Tuned In, and you can too. We invite you to take this journey with us. Be blessed and challenged as you read!

—*Dr. Beverly Rodgers*

We all love our tech—me included. Who doesn't love having a world of information, education, and entertainment right in the palms of our hands? And if it weren't for the GPS function on my phone, I would be wandering aimlessly on some forgotten hillside. I can get lost in a parking lot! As a pastor and counselor, however, my growing concern over the last decade has been the obsession with the digital world that is robbing people of real life that is playing out right in front of them. It's the couples who come to counseling who are drifting apart because they would rather gaze at their phones than each other. It's the epidemic of anxiety in people who check their devices every minute for fear they will miss some news, either good or bad. It's the families who sit down at the dinner table and miss valuable talk-time with each other as they separately scroll through updates on people they barely know. If we don't have the time to disconnect from our digital lives to connect with each other, we certainly won't find time to idle down and connect with the deeper layers of our souls—and with God. Without the strength, hope, and peace that He provides, we can find it impossible to feel anything but anxious and disconnected.

As my concerns grew, I talked to my therapist sister, Bev, to see if this was just a West Coast phenomenon, or if she was experiencing the same thing in her counseling office in the buckle of the Bible belt in North Carolina. Bev is the most compassionate and capable counselor I know. Her heart to help people is matched only by her desire to constantly learn new ways to empower them, as you will discover in all of the up-to-date research included in this project.

When we realized we were witnessing the same dysfunction, we decided to collaborate on this book, not just to sound the warning of too much tech, but to engage readers in the beauty of connecting with a capable God.

The Lord brought Bev and me out of a home filled with anger and abuse and guided us to lives of peace and fulfillment, and we want to show others how to find that abundant life as well. We pray that as you read, you will recognize that God is the God of quirks and quarks, that He can handle calm and chaos, and that He wants you to know He loves you with an unquenchable love. Find Him in the pages of this book as you move from Tech-Pecked to Tuned In.

—*Pastor Linda Newton*

## Chapter 1

# Tech-Pecked, but Tenderhearted

Eric, a self-made man in his late thirties, clearly planned his work and worked his plan. He pursued a relentless agenda, and he made sure everyone knew not to get in his way. Between his work emails and media connections, his workday never seemed to end. For the third time in a week, he wandered into the house from work after dark with his face pasted to his iPhone.

"You're late," his wife, Laurie, reacted, trying not to relay the contempt she was feeling.

"I just got your text, but I figured I would be home soon," he responded, formulating his defense. "I was starving, so I hit the drive-through around the corner from work."

"You didn't eat lunch?" his wife questioned.

"I worked through lunch," Eric responded, still in defense mode, and knowing full well that he had spent his lunch hour on Facebook.

This wasn't the first time Eric had scrolled down a wormhole of information on a social media site before he realized that his entire lunch break was over. He continued to tell Laurie, and anyone who would listen, that he had to be on Facebook because his presence on social media helped to build his business; he was grooming relationships for possible referrals from his online friends. But at his core, Eric worried that he would miss out on the rush he got from viewing the latest post or pic on his newsfeed. And what really gave him a thrill was posting all the awards he received at work and seeing all the "Likes" from his friends, some of whom he had never actually met. On the many nights he spent diving into black holes following the latest news and information online, he discovered articles about tech addictions, but he dismissed the information because nearly everyone he knew lived tech-obsessed. "If I've got a problem, so does the entire free world," he rationalized.

"We waited on dinner as long as we could. The boys had things they wanted to show you. That's why I texted you," Laurie responded, biting her lip to keep from crying.

"Time got away from me. I figured I'd be home right away, so I didn't need to text back," Eric offered absentmindedly, his head still cocked, staring at his screen. In an effort to appease her, he offered, "I'm not hungry, but I can sit here while you eat."

"What's the point if you're going to be on your phone the entire time?" Laurie had reached the end of her patience. "From the moment you step through the door, your face is glued to a screen. Your idea of spending quality time with the kids is to park them in front of a cartoon on Netflix while you check your email.

"The boys and I want you to be with us," Laurie implored. "Your son got an award for being the only six-year-old to jump off the high-dive today, and he couldn't wait to show it to you. He actually came to me crying, asking, 'Is Daddy going to care about us today?' I've never said a word about my frustration to this child. This came directly from him. What must be going on in his young mind to ask a question like that? Jason isn't the only one who feels second fiddle, Eric. Your phone gets more strokes than I do! Every night I leave you sitting on the sofa with a blue glare in your face as you say, 'Just another couple of minutes.' And you wonder why you toss and turn all night when you do finally come to bed. I wouldn't say this if we didn't want you to be in our lives. I've tried; I've pled; I've prayed; and I've cried. I don't know what else to do. The kids are growing up, you are missing it, and it's killing me to watch this happen."

That launched Eric into a defensive diatribe about how hard he had to work to keep his position in the company. "I am doing this for you and the kids," Eric protested. "It takes a lot to stay on top of things. I've explained to you that I have to keep my phone on for the business. There are calls I have to take. I work hard for this family, and I could use a little respect, a little appreciation."

"I let you know every chance I get how much we appreciate you," Laurie pleaded. Deep inside, Eric knew his wife could always be counted on to praise him and the kids, but he felt too proud and too defensive to let her know that in the moment. He continued to defend his position for a few more minutes, until his phone pinged a call. Laurie shrugged her shoulders in hopeless resignation as she climbed the stairs to bed.

Eric and Laurie recycled this same argument at least once a week, and nothing changed until his wife grew tired of playing second fiddle and eventually walked out, taking the kids with her. His tech-pecked lifestyle that compelled him to "connect with people" was alienating him from the people he cared about most. Now it was desperation, not desire, that drove Eric to my (Linda's) counseling office. He had never been to a counselor before, so despite his need to seem in control, his body language betrayed him and displayed his discomfort.

"Don't get me wrong. I love my wife and kids, and I don't want her to go, but she wants so much from me," he stated, fidgeting as he talked. "I don't think she realizes how much work it takes to keep the business going. The minute I look away, everyone stops working and nothing gets done. I've had to make things happen since I was fifteen."

He leaned in to make his point. "I might not be husband of the year, but I'm not nearly as bad as my old man. He was an angry alcoholic. He'd come home drunk and use whoever was in his way as a punching bag, and a lot of the time it was me. His dad, my grandpa, left me fifty grand for college. But before I was old enough to drive, my drunken dad had squandered it all at the local casino. I decided right then, 'If it's going to be, it's up to me!' That has been my motto ever since."

Eric has some deep Soul Wounds that stem from unmet needs from childhood. If not recognized and dealt with, they can affect us in our adult relationships. These wounds cause people to react in unhealthy ways because a past hurt is being triggered and they don't even know it. Eric had vowed not to be his father, but this blinded him to his own unhealthy adaptations.[1]

Eric's candor in the session was unexpected. He was on a roll, and I wasn't stopping him.

"Then I put myself through college, working day and night to make it happen, and became the youngest person to ever fill this position in the history of the company. Laurie said she loved my drive and determination when we met. Now all she's done for the past two years is complain, 'The kids and I never see you, and when you are home, your mind is someplace else or you're in a foul mood or both. We barely see your face. It's always in your phone. We're forgetting what you look like.'"

"My phone is a tool for work, and so is my computer. I can't do my job without them. Can't she see that I am doing all of this for her and the kids? My boys aren't going to have to work like I did. I want them to have what I never had. What does she want from me anyway?" he asked, not expecting an answer.

"I believe it's *you* she wants," I responded, affirming that he was a good guy, one that his family would want to be around. "None of the money, security, or perks matter if she doesn't have the guy she fell in love with."

"You sound like her," he remarked, trying to use humor to deflect the hurt his face was portraying, while dancing away from his real issues.

"Eric, you're an admirable, hardworking man who cares about his family enough to move way out of your comfort zone to come to counseling to figure out what to do save your marriage. No wonder you're the guy your wife wants to spend time with," I reassured him.

---

1: Beverly and Tom Rodgers, *Soul Healing Love*, (Virginia: Selah Publishing, 1998).

"But if you spend all of your time with your face in your phone, no one, not your wife or your kids, get to benefit from all you have to offer. Everyone misses out, including you. It's plain to see that you are working as hard as you can."

"You're right about that. I am working hard," he responded, grateful for my affirmation. "But this is honestly one of the hardest things I've ever done. It's like my devices are somehow calling me to them."

"It's plain to see that you are trying hard and feeling like you are not making the progress you want. Some things in life—in fact, many things in life—we can't do alone. We need help, maybe even divine help.

"This is where faith comes in," I offered. "When we've done the best we can, we can rely on a power greater than ourselves to fill in the gaps. If I go through life feeling like it's all up to me, I'll be exhausted and ill-tempered by noon!"

"Listen, Linda, I'm not going to be one of those 'pray-about-it' types. God helps those who help themselves. Besides, I think people only regurgitate what they have learned as kids. I learned to take care of myself."

"I'm afraid that I am going to put a hole in your theory," I challenged. "I didn't learn about God in my home when I was a kid. In fact, I was ten years old before I realized God's last name didn't start with a *D*."

My honesty and vulnerability clearly captured his attention. Eric needed a change in his life, but he had no idea how much peace and satisfaction he would get from the change. He just knew he was ready.

## Making It Real

1. Does anyone in your life complain that they can't seem to pull your attention away from your digital devices?
2. Do you think their concern is valid? Be honest.
3. If so, write out three things you can you do about it.

4. Eric was struggling to trust God because, since childhood, he had had no one to depend on but himself. Can you relate to his struggle? Why? Why not?

5. When it comes to relying on God on a daily basis, what holds you back from trusting Him? Look at the list below and check which ones apply.

   • Fearing He won't be there if you ask?

   • Fearing you won't like what He wants from you?

   • A habit of self-sufficiency?

   • Misunderstanding His nature?

   • Feelings of unworthiness?

   • Unfamiliarity with His desire to help?

   • How would your life be better if you could trust God in these areas?

6. Ask the Lord to help you identify your hesitance and to help you repair it. Read Philippians 2:13: "For it is God who works in you to will and to act according to his good purpose" (NIV). God will not only give us His divine help, He will also give us the want-to. When we don't have the desire to seek Him, He can even provide that.

Chapter 2

# This Is Your Brain on Tech

As Eric sat drumming his fingers against his thigh and furrowing his brow with apprehension, I asked him, "What if I told you that I have scientific research demonstrating the detriments of too much tech time, and even more research about how you can benefit from prayer?" As a forthright man, he seemed as if he would appreciate a let's-get-down-to-business approach.

"I told myself when I came here that I would be open. It's worked for me in business. So, I'll look at your information, but don't think I'm going to 'get religion' or anything," came his guarded response.

"No worries. I don't believe that it's religion you need," I responded, knowing that it was relationship, not religion, that would make the difference in his life.

I decided to tackle his tech-obsession before we plunged into the God issue. Neither would be easy, but if I could get a buy-in from him on the tech data, then I might have an easier time getting him to receive the prayer research.

## Present in Your Presence

To help him move from tech-wrecked to tech-checked, I started with current research from Dr. Emma Seppala's book, *The Happiness Track: How to Apply the Science of Happiness to Accelerate Your Success*. With the words *happiness* and *success* in the title, I knew he would be tracking with me on its benefits. Her research is beneficial for any of us in the technological age as we struggle to keep up with all of our digital distractions. Have you ever been sitting in a meeting at work when your phone dings with an Instagram update and you find yourself struggling to keep your mind on what the boss is saying? Perhaps your intent is to talk to your kids or your spouse about their day, but you can't resist catching up on the latest news from your five hundred Facebook friends? Maybe you're the culprit who tweets about the lunch you are supposed to eat to your almost-friends on Twitter rather than being present at the table with the friend who invited you to share a meal.[1]

Dr. Seppala states, "That 'multitasking,' instead of helping us accomplish more things faster, actually keeps us from doing anything well. Paradoxically, slowing down and focusing on what is happening in front of you right now—being present instead of always having your mind on the next task to be accomplished—will make you more successful. Research shows that remaining present will make you more productive and happier and, moreover, will give you that elusive quality we attribute to the most successful people: charisma."[2]

Psychologists Matthew Killingsworth and Daniel Gilbert of Harvard University did a study of 5,000 people, stating that adults spend only about 50 percent of their time in the present moment. In other words, they are mentally checked out half the time. Not only did they measure when people's minds were wandering, but the scientists collected information on happiness levels. They found that when we are in the present moment, we are also our happiest, no matter what we are doing. The reason is because we can fully experience the things going on around us. Instead of getting caught up in the race to accomplish more things faster, we slow down and are actually with the people we are with, immersed in the ideas being discussed, and fully engaged in our projects.

---

1 Emma Seppala, "Down With Multitasking: Increase Productivity (and Charisma) by Mastering Singular Focus," *Stanford Medicine Center for Compassion And Altruism Research And Education,* July 30, 2016: http://ccare.stanford.edu/press_posts/down-with-multitasking-increase-your-productivity-and-charisma-by-mastering-singular-focus/
2 Seppala, ibid.

According to Seppala, by being in the present, you will enter a state of flow that is highly productive and you will become charismatic, making the people around you feel understood and supported. You will have good relationships, which are one of the biggest predictors of success and happiness. She is not the only researcher on this bandwagon.[3]

## Switch Cost

Dr. Earl Miller, a professor of neuroscience at Massachusetts Institute of Technology, has done extensive research on what multitasking does to the brain. Miller states, "Every time you switch your focus from one thing to another, there's something called a 'switch-cost.' Your brain stumbles a bit, and it requires time to get back to where it was before it was distracted."

One recent study found that it can take your brain fifteen to twenty minutes to get back to where it was after stopping to check an email. And Miller's own research shows that you don't get better at this sort of multitasking with practice. "In fact, people who judged themselves to be expert digital multitaskers tended to be pretty bad at it," he says. "You're not able to think as deeply on something when you're being distracted every few minutes," Miller adds. "And thinking deeply is where real insights come from."[4]

## Dealing with Distractions

New research shows that merely having to deal with distractions can be harmful. If you are focusing on a boring sales report for work and Pinterest is calling your name, or a text message pings a Facebook update, resisting the urge to respond can have consequences for your brain. Neuroscientist Dr. Adam Gazzaley of the University of California, San Francisco, found that when people try to ignore distractions, it requires significant effort from the brain's prefrontal

---

3 Emma Seppala, "The Secrets of a Happier Life," *The Science of Happiness, Time Special Edition*, October 20, 2018, 13.
4 Markham Heid, "You Asked: Are My Devices Messing With My Brain?" *Time,* May 13, 2015: http://time.com/3855911/phone-addiction-digital-distraction/

cortex. This area is the executive function of our brains, the area that is required for problem-solving, memory, and focus. If most of our mental energy is preoccupied with trying to resist interruptions, our capacity to think deeply and creatively on tasks that require concentration like schoolwork, sales presentations, and other necessary and important goals, is impeded.[5] That says nothing about the concentration needed for the more epic tasks that are built upon the simpler ones. It begs the question, "How would Bach, Einstein, or Thoreau have fared in the technological age?" They might have had more tricks and tools at their disposal with tech devices, but would they have been able to access their creative genius under the onslaught of constant digital interruptions? Not only does multitasking hinder our concentration, but digital dependence can foster unwanted and unsuspected anxiety.

## The Anxiety Epidemic

Dr. Larry Rosen, professor emeritus at California State University, Dominguez Hills, who researches the cognitive effects of digital technology, teamed up with Dr. Gazzaley, mentioned earlier, to write *The Distracted Mind*. Dr. Rosen links smartphones with the growing anxiety epidemic in our culture today. In a blog post for *Psychology Today*, he quotes one study in which participants completed puzzles while an experimenter either called their cell phone (sitting on a table behind them) or did not call their phone. Those who endured the missed call showed increased anxiety, as well as decreased performance on the puzzles compared to a group with no interruption. Another study indicated that even the "mere presence of one's phone led to decreased performance on all but the easiest tasks."[6]

To be in the moment and muffle the multitasking monster, researchers advocate setting limits on our tech use. They recommend setting a time every day, especially when you are with your family, to disconnect.

---

5 *Nir Eyal and Chelsea Robertson, PhD*, "Your Ability to Focus Has Probably Peaked: Here's How to Stay Sharp," *Nir & Far*: https://www.nirandfar.com/.../your-ability-to-focus-has-probably-peaked-heres-how-t...

6 Larry D. Rosen, Ph.D., "Our Social Media Obsession," *Psychology Today*, July 18, 2014: https://www.psychologytoday.com/us/blog/rewired-the.../our-social-media-obsession

I laid out a plan to help Eric live tech-checked not tech-wrecked.

"Buy a watch," I instructed, "not a smart watch, simply one that tells you the time, so that you won't get sucked into the web when you only need to know what time it is. Turn off your phone; mute your alerts, alarms, and ringers for at least two hours in the evening. Then you can be present in your presence. Set specific times every day to answer emails, say noon and four p.m. This puts you in charge of your schedule and not at the beck and call of every ping, ding, or buzz."

Maybe you don't have the freedom in your schedule that Eric did. If you work for someone else and must be available all day long, business must surely be contained within business hours. If that can't happen, show your boss these studies. If he or she still insists on owning your soul, find another job for the sake of your sanity and relationships. Seriously! Of course, this can be hard, but most people like Eric don't realize that being tech-pecked can take its toll on your life and relationships, and this is a serious matter.

The phone is a tool, and tools need to work for you, not the other way around. You get to run your day rather than have it run you. Most of all, you get to be with those people who really care about you. I am betting that most of your friends on Facebook won't show up at your funeral, nor will they cry if you die. But the people right in front of you will never forget you—your kindness and investment, or your lack of it.

It was challenging enough to encourage Eric to wean himself off of his tech-pecked continuous digital dependence, but inspiring him to pray and tune in to God would take some divine intervention. So, I asked the Lord to use my words to speak to his heart. (No surprise that I would employ prayer to motivate someone to pray.) Eric clearly needed to understand the benefit of connecting with God, and how it would free him from his need to depend only on himself. If prayer could help him "let go and let God," he had a better chance of gaining balance in his life. Then he could find time for family and fun. He could embrace the abundant life Christ was offering him and experience the peace he desperately needed.

## Making It Real

1. Take inventory of how many times you check your digital devices every day.

2. Set a goal to turn off your alerts so that you won't be at their mercy, but rather you will be in charge of your moments. Put your phone facedown when you are in meetings or turn it off during movies or church services.

3. How hard or easy is this for you to do?

4. Ask those whom you are close to if you are "present in your presence" when you are with them. Let them speak into your life without getting defensive, and make the necessary changes to be more attentive to those who depend on you.

5. How does it feel to be more in the moment when you are with people? Do they respond to you differently when you are tuned in to them?

6. Decide to live tech-checked by turning your phone off for two hours in the evening and especially during meals. Engage family members in fun and meaningful conversation while you are at the table. We will offer more tools for healthy family time later in this book.

Chapter 3

# This Is Your Brain on Prayer

As often happens, scientific research proves what the Scripture has taught us for years. The front page of *Parade* magazine displayed an article titled, "Why Prayer Could Be Good Medicine." *Parade* was a section of the Sunday newspaper that subscribers looked forward to each week. This was back in the days when people still sat down with a hard copy and a cup of coffee for a leisurely read, unlike now, when we swipe as fast as we can to read as much information as possible in the shortest amount of time.

## The Health Benefits of Prayer

Dr. Harold Koenig, currently the director of Duke University's Center for Spirituality, Theology, and Health, stated: "Prayer—whether for oneself (petitionary prayer) or others (intercessory prayer)—affects the quality if not the quantity of life. It boosts morale, lowers agitation, loneliness and life dissatisfaction and enhances the ability to cope in men, women, the elderly, the healthy and the sick."[1]

The same article noted a study by Dr. Andy Newberg of the University of Pennsylvania in which he documented changes in the blood flow in particular regions of the brain during prayer and

---

1 Diane Hales, "Why Prayer Could Be Good Medicine," *Cengage* https://www.cengage.com/custom/enrichment_modules.bak/data/Why_Prayer_Could_be_Good_Medicine_Hales_Parade.pdf

meditation. He stated, "This could be the link between religion and health benefits such as lower blood pressure, slower heart rates, decreased anxiety and enhanced sense of well-being."

Dr. Newberg was quoted again in *Psychology Today*. He monitored brain activity with a Single Photon-Emission Computed Tomography or SPECT, a device similar to a CAT or PET scan machine. Newberg, along with his colleague, Eugene D' Aquili, observed a decreased level of activity particularly in the orientation association area (OAA) of the brain, the part of the brain responsible for enabling people to distinguish between themselves and objects in the outside world. For doctors Aquili and Newburg, this indicated that "spiritual experience, at its very root, is intimately interwoven with human biology. That biology, in some way, compels the spiritual urge." Or, as others have put it, human brains are wired for God.[2]

There are those who dispute Newberg's work, as they seek to stimulate those very sections of the brain Newberg identified in order to create a religious experience! They may be able to duplicate the euphoric, otherworldly state, but that is only a part of prayer. Getting to know a benevolent God, through the practice of talking to Him regularly, builds trust in an all-powerful heavenly Father who is constantly watching out for His kids.

While these compelling articles managed to impress my skeptical counselee, Eric, I knew that the frustrations about embracing faith were not purely intellectual. Often in my counseling office I encounter people who are angry with the very God in whom they have chosen not to believe! It's quite a contradiction to hold a grudge against someone who doesn't exist, isn't it? But I find that people who share this view are harboring some resentment toward God for the pain they have experienced. It's easier to proclaim God isn't there than it is to try to understand why He didn't protect them from some hurtful situation.

I learned early on that people don't care how much you know until they know how much you care. I care deeply for people with

2 Michael Shermer, Paul Chance, "God on the Brain," *Psychology Today,* June 9, 2016, https://www.psychologytoday.com/us/articles/200111/god-the-brain

painful pasts because I've been there too. I wanted Eric to know he wasn't alone in his struggle. As he sat in my office, I shared the story of where I came from, and how my sister and I survived the roller-coaster ride of my mom's rage and abuse. Eric leaned in and listened. It was a story he could relate to all too well.

## Our Story

For some people, the South conjures up visions of front porch swings, magnolia blossoms, and the faint scent of wisteria. I only wish. For me (Linda), it brings memories of anger, abandonment, abuse, and the smell of stale cigarette smoke. I was one of those kids from a broken home, and I always felt broken.

I never remember praying as a family when I was a kid. There was no grace said at the table, no bedtime prayers offered up for security and safety. In fact, there were very few kind words spoken at all. Most days were filled with contention, criticism, and chaos.

Our dad left when I was five, making my angry mom even angrier. Mama had no problem taking out her rage on her kids. She often said, "If that *expletive* father of yours hadn't left me with four kids, I could have done something with my life."

I thought that, as a mother, she was doing something with her life, but apparently I wasn't important enough to count. If I wasn't the object of her anger, I was filled with guilt because that meant either my twin sister, Bev, or one of my brothers received her wrath. If she woke up in a foul mood for any reason, which happened a lot, fists would fly.

To make ends meet, Mama took a dinner shift waiting tables at a nearby restaurant. That left us kids on our own at night. With my mom yelling obscenities at all hours and her kids running ragged all evening, it's clear that Tennessee trailer trash would have been a step up for us. We were the half-raised heathens that mothers warned their kids to stay away from. And most folks did just that, except for one neighbor from across the street, Mrs. Gober—Maude Gober! How's that for a good Southern name?

Mrs. Gober braved the no-man's-land of our front yard and invited our family to church. She brought Juicy Fruit gum and chocolate cupcakes with pink icing. Bev and I decided that this lady peddling sweets couldn't be all bad. So, we took her up on her offer.

Despite all you hear today about Christians being judgmental, the people in that neighborhood church were anything but. They wrapped their arms around us and made us feel like we belonged. So, we made our way through those church doors every chance we could.

Those caring folks always seemed genuinely glad to see us. Unlike my mom, they didn't treat us like a bother; they treated us like a blessing. Mort Collins had butterscotch candy waiting for us every time we walked through the doors. My Sunday school teachers took an interest in us, making sure I got to church if Mrs. Gober couldn't take us. It was Reverend Laxton, a retired pastor, who bought both my sister and me our very first brand-new Holy Bibles. The folks in that church loved us until we realized Jesus did too.

Then on a hot and sticky summer Sunday in June, I made my way down the aisle of that little country church, and I gave my heart to Christ. At that moment I felt God's love washing over me. I felt His peace and the strength I needed to survive my dysfunctional home life. As I prayed, I recognized that Jesus had paid a price for my past, and His commitment to me brought profound purpose to my life. Through my tears, I looked beside me and there was Bev. She was giving her heart to Jesus too. We became more than sisters that day. We now had an incredible bond in Christ, and we had no idea all God had in store for two damaged girls from a dysfunctional home.

The faithful folks in church became our family. Several of the older ladies came to pray with us that day. After that, any time we asked, they would offer a prayer for us. We never told them how bad things were at home. We knew that would only enrage our mother more. Plus, we didn't want any of these good-willed people to be pulled into the vortex of Mama's drama. Their example of love for God and love for us inspired us to nurture a relationship with God like they had. They were peace-filled women, and we needed some of that peace ourselves.

As I learned to come close to God, there were moments when I sat in God's presence that I felt wrapped up in a blanket of security and transported to a place of unexplainable peace, in spite of the truth that nothing in my world warranted that. When Mama got on her rage-filled rolls, I'd whisper a prayer to not go crazy in the midst of those maddening moments. I could escape on my knees, idle down, and find calm in the midst of the chaos. Bev and I would pray with each other and for each other, and every time we did, it helped us know God better and trust Him more. I shudder to think of where we would have ended up if we hadn't found the Lord.

Because of the difference that reaching out to God made in my everyday life, I now encouraged Eric to give it a try. "The best thing I can offer you is my own experience, strength, and hope. As a pastoral counselor, I have offered this advice many times. If prayer doesn't work, what have you lost? Just talk to God like you're talking to me. You can even tell Him you're not sure about this whole process. I have found that I can tell God how I am feeling, and my frustration doesn't push Him off the throne! Plus, He's God. He already knows what we're thinking anyway.

"If you can connect with God, then you won't have to go it alone every day, will you?" I continued. "And if you discover there is a higher power working for your good, you can relax and know it's not all up to you, can't you?"

Eric nodded pensively, still not sure about all I was presenting.

"I'm not asking you to become a holy-roller, just to try praying. Tell God what you're feeling and what you need. You did come to a Christian counselor. You had to know I would suggest connecting with God as an option," I said with a smile.

"I can't say I'm surprised," he admitted. "But my brother-in-law highly recommended you, and he wasn't going to let up on me until I made this appointment."

"Does that mean you will give God a try? You can blame your brother-in-law and me if nothing happens," I commented, still smiling.

"Okay," came his reluctant reply.

## Eric's Insight

Eric showed up for his next appointment with a mixture of skepticism and surprise.

"I have to tell you, Linda, that I was more than a little frustrated and skeptical when I left your office last week, but something kept repeating our conversation in my head. I decided that I had nothing to lose that wasn't already gone and everything to gain in giving your advice a chance, so I cautiously tried it. Inside I was pretty sure nothing would happen. So, I just said out loud before I went to bed, 'Okay, God, You're supposed to know how I'm feeling, so I don't need to tell You. I don't want to lose my family, but I guess You know that too. If You are really there, can You help me out?' I said I would try praying, and I did. Then I just rolled over and went to sleep.

"I woke up feeling no different, just as I had suspected, but for some reason I decided to call my wife. She hadn't been taking my calls, so I wasn't even sure she would answer. Still, something nagged me to call. It had been weeks since we talked, but this time she picked up and she didn't hang up. I got to tell her about our appointment, and I shared some of the research you gave me, at least what I could remember of it. I even told her about my prayer. I let her know that I could change and that I would change. The life I was living wasn't just making her crazy, it was making me nuts too. It took her leaving for me to see that. I don't want to live life without Laurie or my kids. Honestly, I was surprised she stayed on the phone because she seemed so determined that we were over when she left.

"Laurie told me that she had been praying for our marriage for years. She said, 'I've never stopped loving you, and that's why your preoccupation with everything but us hurts me so much.' That was hard to hear, Linda. But you'll be proud of me. I didn't get defensive, I just listened. We were on the phone for three hours that night! It pains me to realize that we haven't talked that long or that deeply since we were first married. I'm starting to recognize what I have been missing out on in our relationship, not to mention what I've missed out on with the boys.

"She reluctantly agreed to go to dinner with me that Friday, but I had to promise I would be on my best behavior (no defensive anger, excuses, or justifications) and that it would be not be a tech-pecked evening. I kept my promise, but it was a challenge. It was hard because I got four calls that evening, but I kept my phone in my pocket so I wouldn't answer it. I have to be honest. When you started talking about being 'tech-pecked,' as you call it, I thought you were dead wrong. But as I sat there with Laurie, the love of my life, someone I do not want to lose, and actually struggled not to answer my phone, I realized I have a problem.

"When I got home, I could see that all four of the calls could have waited. And they did! I'm learning," Eric offered, with a look of relief.

"Laurie told me she was shocked in a good way that I didn't look at my phone the entire night. Sadly, she said she couldn't remember the last time that had happened. Neither could I.

"Before the night was over, Laurie thanked me for calling her, and especially for not answering my cell when it buzzed. Then she thanked me for praying. She said it was something she has always wanted me to do. It wasn't until then that I understood that God had actually heard me and answered my prayer. I know that Laurie is nowhere near ready to come home, but I feel like after our good talk there just may be hope for us."

A simple prayer prayed with barely any faith brought an answer to Eric's prayer. That inspired him to take a closer look at what a relationship with God could offer him. In his words, "I wasn't doing so hot on my own, so asking for God's help was worth a try."

## Making It Real

1. Try taking a tech break from your devices and see what happens. Decide not to be tech-pecked for an hour, maybe two, perhaps an entire evening. Write about how you feel.
2. Have you, like Eric, chosen to take a tech break from your phone only to find that the calls you missed weren't as critical as you thought?

3. Ask yourself if the calls you missed were as urgent as you once thought. If not, write what you think about this realization.

4. Take a moment to quiet your soul or to spend quality time with face-to-face, real-live people right in front of you.

5. Dr. Harold Koenig's research about prayer states, "It boosts morale, lowers agitation, loneliness and life dissatisfaction and enhances the ability to cope in men, women, the elderly, the healthy and the sick." Have you ever experienced any of these benefits as you engaged in prayer? Journal about your experience.

6. Eric's approach to God in prayer was cavalier at best and disrespectful at worst. Yet God still answered his prayers. What does this demonstrate to you about the nature of God?

7. As you think about God intervening in Eric's life in a miraculous way, translate this into your own faith journey. Do you see a pattern of God's care and provision, i.e., bringing people at just the right time, engineering circumstances, closing doors, and opening others? Write about how you see God's intervention in your life.

8. Pray for someone with whom you can share that story in the next few days. If you are still waiting for an answer from the Lord, pray that someone will inspire you with their story.

Chapter 4

# Actual versus Virtual

In a moment of desperation, Eric was willing to give God a try, and it paid off. But to sustain an actual, viable relationship with a caring God, prayer needs to become a daily priority. It isn't just reserved for when we are in trouble or when we want the Lord to do something for us. It is an ongoing dialogue with the everlasting God. It is as simple as talking to God and as complex as talking to God! It's a natural process with supernatural results.

Jesus knows what we need before we ask, but when we speak out our need to a personal God, it lifts our burdens from us. When we present them to Him, it opens up heaven and brings His power to us. That brings us to the **3A's**: For an A+ Connection with God: Ask, Acknowledge, and Align. The first is to **Ask**.

## Ask

God invites us to connect with Him through the amazing privilege of prayer. We can't partner with Him unless we embrace the practice. When we approach Him, it's okay to ask for what we need. Jesus said in Matthew 7:7–8, "Ask and it will be given to you; seek and you will find; knock and the door will be opened to you. For everyone who asks receives; the one who seeks finds; and to the one who knocks, the door will be opened" (NIV).

Jesus was explaining to a crowd the all-encompassing favor God has for His children so He chose the most obvious example of unconditional love He had available: the parent/child relationship. "You parents—if your children ask for a loaf of bread, do you give them a stone instead? Or if they ask for a fish, do you give them a snake? Of course not! So if you sinful people know how to give good gifts to your children, how much more will your heavenly Father give good gifts to those who ask him" (Matthew 7:9–11 NLT).

I (Beverly) remember when Linda and I were just learning about the new Bibles that a retired pastor in church had given us. Our youth pastor, Richard Smith, stood up to teach and said, "Let's turn to Matthew 7:9." I was new to finding books in the Bible, so I started my slow search. With my head buried in my beautiful new Bible with its crisp pages, Richard started to speak: "Which of you if your son asks for bread, will give him a stone?" I was deep in my search and not focusing, so I actually thought that Richard was asking a question. In response I raised my hand to give him an affirmative answer.

"Beverly," he questioned, "why did you raise your hand?"

Somewhat distracted from my search and a bit confused, I said, "Well, you asked who would give your kid a stone if they asked for bread, and my answer is my mom just might, depending what kind of mood she was in that day."

Sweet Richard looked at me with compassion and gently explained that he wasn't asking a question, he was merely reading from the Scripture. He was so gentle I wasn't even embarrassed. But I did realize, as did many of the people in the room at the time, that I had a deep feeling of lovelessness from my mom. It took time to heal that soul wound, and prayer was a great part of the remedy.

For those of us whose parents didn't give us good gifts like Jesus referenced, our trust in God has to be built as we continue to ask and find Him trustworthy.

James 4:2 tells us, "You do not have because you do not ask God" (NIV). Jesus explains that God wants to answer us, but He has something to say about how to ask: "When you are praying, do not heap up empty phrases as the Gentiles do; for they think they will be heard because of their many words. Do not be like them, for your Father knows what you need before you ask him" (Matthew 6:7–8 ESV). I am not sure what "empty phrases" the Gentiles in Jesus' day might have used, but today we have our own problems, according to Pastor John Gaston. He identifies some prayer styles that we employ: The "Call 9-1-1" prayer: This is the "God, I've got an emergency" prayer.

Such prayers are considerate about not wanting to clutter God's schedule on His busy days. They are based on the idea that we should not trouble Him unless it's an emergency. God is essentially a divine spare tire, according to this kind of prayer.

The "Jiminy Cricket" approach: "When you wish upon a star, makes no difference who you are, anything your heart desires will come to you." This views God as a cosmic grandpa who will give you anything that you want.

The "Aladdin's Lamp" prayer: This approach is based on the belief that if you just "rub" God the right way, He might magically be at your service. God is treated like a cosmic bellhop.

The "Lottery" approach: This approach assumes that it can't hurt to try to pray, and you just might hit the jackpot.

The "Guinness" prayer: *Long* is the idea here—and sometimes loud. Those using this approach are trying to win the *Guinness Book of World Records* in their prayer lives. They might pray all night and perhaps wear down God's resistance, or maybe they think He just didn't understand their request at the first mention. Followers of this approach can't forget the story about that widow who kept begging and finally got her request.[1]

## Prayer Is Not Begging

I (Beverly) suffered from what I call "longing prayers," or, more accurately, "whining prayers." Lacking faith in a caring God, I would whine and beg rather than asking in a healthy way. As I look back, I now realize that I was asking for something that I wanted, without asking God what He wanted for me. So, like a whining toddler, if I said "*please*" enough, He would relent. In those years, I felt the Lord's

1 John Gaston, "Boldness at the Throne," *Sermon Central*, July 7, 2016, https://www.sermoncentral.com/sermons/boldness-at-the-throne-john-gaston-sermon-on-god-s-nature-202877

patience with me as I learned to model His sacrificial prayer in the garden: "Not My will but Thine (His Father's) be done." If I seek His will, there's no need to whine because I am praying for what He wants and not for my own agenda. While it's hard to do, it creates so much peace.

Even when we know that what we are praying for is God's will, like the salvation of a loved one or for a family member to leave an addiction behind, we can still struggle with the belief that our prayers matter. I (Linda) believe that kind of fear can be fostered in our family of origin. If the world in which you grew up was not a trustworthy place, it's hard to believe that you can count on God—or anyone else, for that matter. So, when I prayed, it came from the perspective of being hurt by life, and my prayer time looked more like a fearful fretting session than calm communication with a caring God. Yet everything I read in His Word told me that God cared about what I asked for. It just failed to make the twelve-inch drop from my head to my heart. So, I asked God to make that happen. (Here I am praying for a better ability to pray. Why not? He wants us to take everything to Him. Right?)

One morning as I opened my Bible, I came across this verse in Micah 7:7: "As for me, I watch in hope for the LORD, I wait for God my Savior; my God will hear me" (NIV). Those words jumped off the page at me. The prophet Micah was standing his ground stating that "as for me," no matter what anyone one else thought or did, he was going to "watch in hope for the Lord, his Savior." The Lord was Micah's Savior, and He certainly was mine too. When I think of all that He has saved me from, it gives me hope that His answers are worth waiting for. His last line of affirmation gave my heart new conviction: "My God will hear me." This verse informs me not to pray out of hurt, but to pray out of hope; not out of fear, but out of faith with the deep conviction that the One who can answer my prayer is listening. Now when my words start to come from that place of fear deep inside me, I recite this verse and find new resolve.

I've learned that prayer isn't the process of pestering God. We don't have to beg; we simply have to ask. He is ready to respond and even give us what we need when we call on Him. Hebrews 4:15–16 tells us, "We don't have a high priest who is out of touch with our reality. He has been through weakness and testing, experienced it all—all but the sin. So let's walk right up to him and get what he is so ready to give. Take the mercy, accept the help" (MSG).

## Yolanda's Story

Yolanda was a heavy-hearted mother who needed the mercy and help this scripture talks about. Her youngest son had just boarded a plane for Arlington, Virginia, leaving her with an empty nest and a mind filled with worries and concerns. She had known the Lord long enough to know that He was trustworthy, but this was her precious son, and he was heading off to be trained for military service during a time of war.

"I fell asleep that night praying for my son and for me—that I could trust God and not worry myself into an early grave," she shared.

"I had to work that Sunday morning, but my soul felt dry and doubting. I needed to go to church. Even though there were only twenty minutes left in the service, I made my way to one of the back rows looking for a seat. I didn't know we were having a guest speaker that day. Just as I sat down, I heard the speaker say that he was in California all the way from Arlington, Virginia! I felt God-bumps up and down my arms.

"The minute the service ended, I headed up the aisle to the speaker, introduced myself, and told him my story. He graciously offered to pray for my son. Then he went one step further. He asked for my son's contact info and offered to help him find a church in town when he arrived."

You can't tell me that was a coincidence. God heard this weary mother's heart, and He was already at work in her son's life. In less than twenty-four hours, her prayers for her son were answered.

## God's Three Answers to Prayer

God readily responded to this burdened mom's request, but what about those folks who ask and ask and can't seem to get the answer they are seeking? Many stop bothering to ask because they don't believe He is a benevolent God who wants to help them, or they grow weary of trying—like Emily.

A pretty woman in her early twenties with fiery brown eyes and a wild streak to match, Emily came to see me (Beverly) for counseling. She was ready to give up because she was dealing with a great deal of anxiety and fear in her life.

As she sat in the lobby outside my office, I noticed her face intent on her phone and her thumbs scrolling while her two-year-old daughter tried desperately to get her attention. It made me sad to see them, because those waiting-room moments had always been precious to me when my kids were little. Now moms feel the urgency to see what the rest of the world is up to. Before the digital age, it was just my child and me. There was nothing on the agenda, so we could explore the world around us. That's when we practiced saying new words or looking at books. I am not patting myself on the back. Rather, I am shouting out a warning to the tech generation. I can't express how much I now *miss* those precious seconds that seemed so insignificant at the time, but they ended up being so cherished later. They can create priceless memories for moms, not to mention to their kids, as they take the time to read, teach, play with, talk to, or just love on them.

For those of us mothers with empty nests, we actually ache for those moments that seemed to vaporize right before our eyes. And we can't get them back, can we? The best we can do now is to invest in our grandkids. But as good as that is, it's not the same. What I am saying is that these quiet moments with little ones need not be sacrificed to social media or to Pinterest, no matter how voraciously these sites call our names. We have to make sure that we aren't trading virtual moments for real ones, that living tech-pecked isn't keeping us from tuning in to our family members, especially our vulnerable children.

As Emily's mom came to get her daughter, she finally put away her phone and slipped into my office to start her session.

"I'm not asking for a lot, Dr. Bev. I don't want a million dollars. I just want a good guy to marry. I have a two-year-old, no job, and no hope of one. I get so bummed that all I do is eat and drink too much on the weekends when I don't have my daughter. I've gained forty pounds in the last year alone," she informed me, frustrated with herself and feeling discouraged. We addressed her anxiety and depression but also looked at her relationship dilemma.

"I need somebody to take care of us, to take us away from here. Things are so bad with my daughter's dad, I just want to move away and not have to deal with him at all. And I am so sick and tired of going on Facebook only to see all of my classmates with beautiful families and lives everyone else wants to have, while here I am flabby, single, and stuck. I'm afraid I'll never have the life I want. I've all but given up on God, and I barely even pray anymore."

There were so many issues to unpack from what this disillusioned young woman had just stated. But before she gave up on prayer and God, whose help she truly needed, I started with her first comment.

"Emily, I can understand your frustration. You keep praying and you're not getting the simple answer you desire. But I believe God has three answers to prayer: 'yes,' 'not now,' and 'I have something better.'

"I have written books for singles and counseled thousands over the past forty years, and I have found that in order for you to attract Mr. Right, you have to become Ms. Right. We have to get you past your depression and disillusionment so that you can see yourself for the attractive lady that you are.

"You stated that you have little to offer a man—a two-year-old whose dad you hate, no job, no income on the horizon, and forty extra pounds that you put on from drinking too much to mask the pain of loneliness and regret. Do you think you are ready for Mr. Right? If he showed up right now, what would he see?"

Emily paused for a moment, dropped head to her chest, and mumbled, "A mess."

I told her that I didn't see a mess. I saw a young woman who had the courage to get help and that although she might feel like a mess now, she was "In Progress."

"Right now, your focus needs to be on providing for yourself and your daughter. You take care of you and let God take care of bringing Mr. Right your way. Besides, a needy woman isn't attractive to anyone, including herself, right?

"You're a beautiful lady with a delightful smile and a wonderful dedication to your daughter," I assured her. "Let's begin the journey of healing—of getting to know and love yourself so that you can experience God's soul-healing love as well. What do you say?"

To my surprise, my young protégé had no excuses. She was ready to cooperate. First, I furnished her with some interesting findings about Facebook users to help her move from tech-wrecked and discouraged to tech-checked and more productive. Here is some of the information I shared with her.

"Emily, you may be surprised to know that frequent Facebook users report a decline in overall satisfaction with life.[2] Facebook is great for keeping up with people who have moved away, and even for connecting with long-lost relatives, but there is a downside. It plays into our human nature and our tendency to constantly compare ourselves with our peers, and even strangers, for that matter. On Facebook, we tend to show the best of how we are living. We want folks to see our new motorhome, but they don't get to see the fight we had about making the payments. You get to see your friend's kids who were all manners and smiles at the zoo, while your own kids were fighting before they even got out of the car. One of your old teammates from college just got the Camaro you have been dreaming of for the past two years. Now, even if you get one, you won't have the bragging rights because he got one first. Your neigh-

---

2 Ethan Kross, Philippe Verduyn, Emre Demiralp, Jiyoung Park, David Seungjae Lee, Natalie Lin, Holly Shablack, John Jonides, Oscar Ybarra, "Facebook Use Predicts Declines in Subjective Well-Being in Young Adults," *Plos One*, August 14, 2013, http://journals.plos.org/plosone/article?id=10.1371/journal.pone.00698

bors just posted pics of their trip to Aruba, while you are packing up the camper for a cheap trip to the woods because you had to replace your plumbing...and the beat goes on.

"Experts widely recommend electronic time-outs, and even email-free Saturdays and Sundays. That can apply to Facebook as well. If we are going to circle the drain every time we go online, perhaps we need to limit the time we spend on social media and do something more uplifting. Being present in the present is a great substitute, replacing our virtual relationships with real ones. Being in the moment with the people right in front of us not only adds value to them, but it fills our own tanks as well. Let Facebook be a condiment, not a main course. Find fulfillment in actual relationships before losing your self-esteem to what you think is going on in the lives of others."

These words made sense to Emily, and the heartache of feeling inferior to so many of her friends compelled her to curb her digital distractions and try to spend more quality time with her young daughter. She even registered for a class at the local junior college on a night when her mother could babysit instead of taking it online, so she could meet more people her age.

The rest of her plan for self-care included soul-healing therapy sessions, an exercise program to boost her norepinephrine, and time for herself. We also worked on tools to help her reconnect with the faith that had once seemed less important than the partying she did in her teen years. To let go of her resentment toward her spiteful, irresponsible ex, she would need supernatural help.

Emily came in regularly for her appointments and worked hard to understand herself and grow. But some issues were harder than others as she moved two steps forward and one step back struggling to change her old patterns of behavior.

"Don't worry; it's persistence, not perfection, we're after," I continued to assure her.

Finding herself impatient with the goals on which we had agreed, she jumped back online full-steam-ahead and signed up for a matchmaking service, even though we had discussed waiting until she had done more work on herself and felt more prepared. It seems that some bad habits are hard to break. During her third contact with Mr. Possible, she went on a rant about her ex, and he suddenly quit emailing her. Hurt and angry, she came to her appointment sobbing.

"I don't know if I'm more angry at myself or Match Number 9," she lamented. "Everyone kept saying I wasn't ready to meet a prospective partner, but I was tired of being alone and feeling bad. I know now they were right. This was a mistake. I didn't know how bad my anger really sounded until I heard it spewing out of my mouth at this perfect stranger who only wanted to meet a 'nice Christian girl.'" She sighed.

"You're not the first person to run ahead of God's plan, Emily," I assured her. "The Bible is full of stories of folks who have done that. Things didn't go too well for them either.

"Let's get back to the plan that we had originally laid out to help you become Ms. Right before we set out to find Mr. Right," I said with a smile. "Focus your prayers on asking God to help you do that, and especially to let go of your resentment, even if your daughter's dad doesn't deserve it. Your job is to keep your side of the street clean."

"Deal," she agreed as she dried her eyes. We spent the rest of the session helping her unpack the deep soul wounds that had contributed to her anger and bitterness so that she could create a life worth enjoying.

Emily's exercise program gave her more confidence, enhanced positive brain chemicals, and empowered her as she enrolled in school. Her classes stimulated her brain, and that helped when she opened the Bible and began to digest more helpful tools. The insight she gained from counseling and from Scripture brought her to a place where she could forgive her ex and move on with her life. After months of hard work, she felt ready to meet someone and date in a healthy way. That was a good thing because several matches in with eharmony, she met Max, a strong Christian with a similar history to hers and an equal desire to move past his past and embrace health.

"He's great, Dr. Bev. He's crazy about me and my daughter, and I think he is awesome. I'm not clingy because I really feel like I have something to offer him. He does too, because he tells me that all the time." She beamed. "I really believe God brought him into my life."

After delighting with her in this new relationship, I reminded her of our first conversation. "Emily, do you remember our first session, when we talked about God's three answers to prayer?"

As a good student of recovery, Emily paid attention and finished my sentence: "'Yes,' 'not now,' and 'I have something better.' I fully believe that if God had answered my prayer and given me a man to rescue my daughter and me before I was ready, the relationship would not have lasted a year. The Lord knew what He was doing with the 'not now' answer at that time. Now I fully believe that Max is the 'I have something better' answer God knew about all along."

"I think you're pretty smart, Ms. Right."

"I'm so glad I waited on God," she confided.

"Me too."

Just then Emily's phone buzzed, and she quickly shut it off as we finished talking. "I forgot to turn off my phone before I came in. I'm still trying to let go of old patterns," she confessed, "but I am far less of an information junkie than when I started counseling."

"Keep it up, girl. I know that all those who love you will appreciate it."

The psalmist David expressed Emily's sentiments best in Psalm 37:23–25: "The Lord directs the steps of the godly. He delights in every detail of their lives. Though they stumble, they will never fall, for the Lord holds them by the hand. Once I was young, and now I am old. Yet I have never seen the godly abandoned or their children begging for bread" (NLT).

Emily's heart toward God changed as she trusted Him enough to ask for what she needed. When we recognize how capable and caring He is and His great power to provide, we can have confidence as we seek Him. He has the ability and the desire to help us. Which brings us to the next A for an A+ connection with God: **Acknowledge**—who He is and how much He has our backs.

## Making It Real

1. Ask yourself if your devices are making you feel anxious as you wait for something to happen.
2. Are they preventing you from being in the moment with the people right in front of you?
3. Purpose in your heart to keep your phone in your pocket during those moments, so that you can create memories. When you open up your phone, ask yourself, "Is there a real relationship I should be investing in instead of a virtual one right now?"
4. Prayer is a simple as talking to God. Talk to Him as comfortably as you would talk to a friend over coffee. Approach God in prayer and ask Him for something your heart desires.
5. As you think about your prayer life, consider this question: Is there something you have wanted to ask God for but you feel too discouraged or afraid to do so? Remember, prayer is as simple as talking to God. Talk to Him as comfortably as you would a friend over coffee. Approach God in prayer and ask Him for your heart's desire.
6. What do you think about God's three answers to prayer: "yes," "not now," and "I have something better"? If God's answer seems to be no to something you desire right now, do you believe He has something better in store for you?
7. How hard is it for you to surrender to God's will and wait for your "something better"? Why? Why not?

8. Write out a prayer asking for God to give you patience to wait for His perfect will for an important situation in your life.

9. Perhaps your parents did not model God's love. What sense of hurt or loss do you feel because of that? Do you have a hard time feeling loved, trusting other people, and/or feeling like you are enough? Speak that out to the Lord and ask Him to heal your hurts. Write out your prayer.

Chapter 5

# Updating Our Software

When our digital devices fail to function properly, we seek to update our software until things are operating at maximum capacity. Most folks seek any and every update in an effort to understand and utilize every asset their tech device provides. It makes sense, doesn't it?

We have grown dependent on our digital devices to keep us current on what is happening all over the world, whether that news stresses us out or not. We rely on technology to provide us with the tools we need for our life choices. If we invest that same effort in learning who God is and continuously "updating" our view of all He has to offer us, then we can learn how to depend on Him for help, hope, and healing. That enables us to build a life-changing trust in His capable care. When we monitor our tech use, we can free up more time for contemplation and searching out the deeper things in life, like opening up God's Word to discover what a real relationship with Him can look like.

Sarah Young writes, "Instead of focusing on fickle, ever-changing news broadcasts, tune in to the living Word—the One who is always the same. Let Scripture saturate your mind and heart, and you will walk steadily along the path of life. Even though you don't know what will happen tomorrow, you can be absolutely sure of your ultimate destination: *'I hold you by your right hand and afterward*

*I will take you to glory.*'" Then she references Psalm 73:23–24, which affirms her italics.[1]

Downloading a continual belief that God is in your corner can be a real challenge as you begin your journey of faith. As girls who grew up in a home filled with anger and abuse, we understand how challenging it can be to acknowledge that a God we can't see wants to take care of us, when the parents we could see didn't.

Perhaps you suffer from a "broken truster" as the folks you were supposed to be able to count on let you down, so now trusting God seems to require more from you than you can muster. To build your trust, you need accurate information about God's nature and time to watch His faithfulness in your life. The best place to learn about God's intentions toward us is by checking out what He says in His Word. In the last chapter we explored the first of our **3 A's:** For an A+ Connection with God: **Ask**. Let's now examine our second A: **Acknowledge.**

## Acknowledge

Jesus instructed His disciples how to pray in Matthew 6:9–10: "Our Father who art in Heaven, hallowed be Thy name. Thy Kingdom come. Thy will be done on earth, as it is in Heaven" (KJ21). I have heard God called an egotist because He needs to be acknowledged as "hallowed," or "holy." He certainly knows who He is, and He doesn't need us to tell Him that. We're the ones who need to be reminded that not only does He listen as He resides in His heaven, but He is the One who created it all. He is a holy God, a perfect God, and He has our best interests at heart.

Acknowledging how powerful He is and how much He cares for each of us builds our confidence that He can help us get through the challenges that life presents.

For the one who needs healing, He is *Jehovah-Rophe*. For the one who needs peace, He is *Jehovah-Shalom*. For the one struggling to survive, He is *Jehovah-Jireh*, Our Provider. He loves us with an unfailing love, and He will take care of us.

1 Sarah Young, *Jesus Calling* (Nashville: Thomas Nelson, 2015), 115.

When we call on Him, God is delighted because we are acknowledging Him and His place in our lives. Luke 12:32 reads, "Do not be afraid, little flock, for your Father has been pleased to give you the kingdom" (NIV). I (Linda) love it when anyone calls me "little"! Because it's God's pleasure to give us the kingdom, we should take Him up on that offer. We can recognize that not only does He want to give us good things, but He's God, and so He can. That can be a hard concept to get our heads around.

## To Whom Do You Pray?

Jeanna was a new believer with a keen mind, and a way of expressing herself that was almost as colorful as her tattoos. She had come into church identifying herself as a "spiritual person," but she wasn't sure about "all of the Jesus talk" she was hearing around her.

"I stayed at first because I was curious. I kept coming back because I really felt like the ladies here cared about me. That hasn't been easy for me to find in my life," she confided to me (Linda) in a quiet moment over coffee.

"The women here loved me when I couldn't love myself," she continued. "That's when I decided that I wanted what they had. It was a trip to have all these old ladies praying for me in church when I went forward for prayer." She grinned.

"Hey, watch it!" I joked. "I was one of those ladies!"

One day after Bible study, Jeanna frankly questioned, "When I pray, to whom am I supposed to pray, Jesus or God? If I am going to acknowledge my higher power, I want it to be the right one. Understanding the Trinity: God, the Father; Jesus, the Son; and the Holy Spirit threatens to eat my brain!"

"I don't want you wandering around here with half a brain," I informed her. "So, I will do my best to answer your question through what Scripture shows us."

Perhaps you have had questions like Jeanna. For answers, we can open up God's Word to see what Jesus Himself had to say. John 14:5–6 reads, "Thomas said to him, 'Lord, we don't know where you are going, so how can we know the way?' Jesus answered, 'I am the way and the truth and the life. No one comes to the Father except through me'" (NIV).

Jesus is saying that it doesn't matter what church we attend, how good we are, or how good we look to the people around us, accepting Him is the path to God.

Christ continues in John 14:7–11 with these words: "If you really knew me, you would know my Father as well. From now on, you do know him and have seen him.'" Philip said, "Lord, show us the Father and that will be enough for us.'" Jesus answered: "Don't you know me, Philip, even after I have been among you such a long time? Anyone who has seen me has seen the Father. How can you say, 'Show us the Father'? Don't you believe that I am in the Father, and that the Father is in me? The words I say to you are not just my own. Rather, it is the Father, living in me, who is doing his work. Believe me when I say that I am in the Father and the Father is in me; or at least believe on the evidence of the miracles themselves" (NIV).

When I read these words, I see the embodiment of God in the person of Jesus. I could pray to either one, because they are different aspects of the same being. The apostle Paul further explains this in the first chapter of Colossians: "Christ is the visible image of the invisible God. He existed before God made anything at all and is supreme over all creation. Christ is the one through whom God created everything in heaven and earth. He made the things we can see and the things we can't see— kings, kingdoms, rulers, and authorities. Everything has been created through him and for him. He existed before everything else began, and he holds all creation together. Christ is the head of the church, which is his body. He is the first of all who will rise from the dead, so he is first in everything. For God in all his fullness was pleased to live in Christ, and by him God reconciled everything to himself. He made peace with everything in heaven and on earth by means of his blood on the cross" (Colossians 1:15–20 NLT).

As I read these words to Jeanna, I found myself humbled, once again, by what they revealed. "God, the Creator of the cosmos, became man in the form of Jesus, who died a criminal's death on the cross for your sins and mine. Nobody ever loved me like that before," I shared with this sincere seeker.

"I know what you mean," Jeanna replied. "I figured that if someone like Him could love someone like me, I'd be a fool not to follow Him."

"I agree with you there, girl. Then there's the words of the apostle Paul, who clarifies the nature of Christ even further in Philippians 2:5–11: 'Have this attitude in yourselves which was also in Christ Jesus, who, although He existed in the form of God, did not regard equality with God a thing to be grasped, but emptied Himself, taking the form of a bond-servant, and being made in the likeness of men. Being found in appearance as a man, He humbled Himself by becoming obedient to the point of death, even death on a cross. For this reason also, God highly exalted Him, and bestowed on Him the name which is above every name, so that at the name of Jesus every knee will bow, of those who are in heaven and on earth and under the earth, and that every tongue will confess that Jesus Christ is Lord, to the glory of God the Father' (NASB).

"Jeanna, while these and other verses helped me to wrap my head around God being made up of a Trinity, it was a sermon delivered by Reverend Miller, that deep-voiced Southern pastor who gave the altar call the day I accepted Jesus as my Savior, that helped me turn a corner in my understanding," I continued to explain to my eager student.

## The Lord Hears

"Since my spiritual gift is making a short story long, here's the long version!"

We both laughed as I continued to expound. "When I made a decision to follow Christ, my mom was less than pleased that her young'uns had 'fallin' in with all those holier-than-thou hypocrites,' one of her many derisive terms for Christians. So, she made every effort to discourage my sister, Bev, and me from going to church. It was Christmastime, and since our family wasn't much for celebration of any kind, we were excited to finally have something special to do at Christmas.

"However, before we could leave for the Christmas Eve service that night, my mom had one of her many monster-mother moments, ranting again about how my dad had left us so she had to work, even on Christmas.

"'If I have to work, you have to work,' she railed, as she stormed through the house listing off all the tasks that we would have to complete before we could go to church. Then she slammed the door to make her point and headed for her dinner shift at a local restaurant. I always felt as though she was so unhappy with her life that she couldn't stand to see anyone else finding any enjoyment.

"After finishing everything on my mother's list, I finally arrived at the service late. I had missed the drama presentation, something I had really looked forward to seeing. I sat in the back so that no one would see the steady stream of tears soaking my face. Bev sat next to me, neither of us speaking, not wanting to concede the constant hurt that was part of every day in our hopeless home.

"'I am trying the best I can,' I prayed. 'But nothing I do makes Mama happy,' I lamented. 'Is it always going to be this hard?' I questioned God just as the pastor came to the pulpit to present his sermon.

"I heard Reverend Miller say, 'On that first Christmas Eve, Jesus, God incarnate, took human form. He came as a baby to a lowly stable, so that the lowly would know that He came for them too. That Baby grew into a Man so He could die on the cross for your sins and mine.'

"In that moment sitting in the service, I had a simple, but profound realization that God came as a man in the form of Jesus with arms that would hold me up when I needed support, with a lap I could crawl up in when life felt overwhelming, and with hands that would hold mine and lead me on a path to sanity and peace. In the quiet of that Christmas Eve service, as the candles flickered and the choir softly sang, I crawled up into Jesus' lap and found comfort.

"Ann Voskamp says it well: 'Our God who cradles whole inking galaxies in the palm of His hand, whom highest heavens cannot contain—He folds Himself into skin, and uncurls His newborn fingers in the cradle of a barn feeding trough...and we are saved from ourselves.'[2]

"That evening and so many after, I have felt saved from myself and I've lost count of the times I rested in Jesus' lap since then. When the Lord said in Matthew 11:28–30, 'Come to me, all you who are weary and burdened, and I will give you rest. Take my yoke upon you and learn from me, for I am gentle and humble in heart, and you will find rest for your souls. For my yoke is easy and my burden is light,' the Creator of the universe was talking to me...and to you—and He's available 24/7, 365 days a year."

"Your spiritual gift isn't just making a short story long," Jeanna informed me. "It's making people cry." She wiped the eye makeup that was running down her cheeks. "That's a great story and something I'll remember when I need to crawl into someone's lap, because I need to do that a lot!"

"You're not alone," I responded. "In answer to your question about to whom we pray, I can make a case for God, our heavenly Father, or for Jesus, the Son who took on human form. Those who are far smarter than me say that the Holy Spirit serves both God and Jesus, so we gain access to Him through God and Christ.

"I didn't have a father in my home from age five, so it comforts me that I can call on my heavenly Father any time. Having a Savior, Jesus, with strong shoulders, open arms, and a welcoming lap, fills my tank as well. And there are times when my prayer is a simple cry for help, and I feel the Holy Spirit filling me as He downloads the fruit of love, joy, peace, and patience that are far beyond my ability to muster on my own. It blows my mind how they are all one in the same. Understanding that is way above my paygrade, but experiencing the benefit to the three-in-one relationship isn't. My need at the moment dictates to whom I pray, but the comfort I receive is always well worth the time invested."

"I'm getting that," Jeanna reported. "The more I spend time offloading my worries to God or opening His Word, the more I feel

---

2 Footnote Ann, Voskamp, *The Greatest Gift* (Carol Stream: Tyndale, 2013), 139.

His peace. My life can be so chaotic that I crave the peace I feel in God's presence.

"Ditto," I affirmed.

As Jeanna and I finished our coffee and conversation, she was pleased to show me the apps that she employed to keep her on track with her Bible reading.[3] I applauded her practicality. She wanted to learn more about God, so applying the tools of our techno-savvy society to achieve that goal was admirable. She was also quick to inform me that she had downloaded an app to keep her accountable for the times when she checked her phone each day. She read my blog posts about the research linking digital demands and anxiety and readily remarked, "I don't want to live so tech-pecked that I miss out on the real moments of life. And besides, I have enough anxiety each day without my cell phone adding to the problem."

Just like Jeanna, we recognize that acknowledging God's nature and abilities has a profound effect on our confidence to call on Him. In the next chapter we will learn about the last of our **3 A's** for an A+ Connection with Christ—**Align**. We can discover an amazing peace when we seek to align with His plans for us, but that is no easy feat with digital demands bombarding our days.

## Making It Real

1. It seems ironic to go online to find apps to curb online use, and even paradoxical to install an app on our phones to keep us from checking them every minute. But we have recommended it to many clients and found that it works. Our phones are always with us. To keep us from obsessing on the stimuli they provide, we can download apps that will help us both monitor our phone use and still use our phones as tools to provide us with relevant devotionals. Check for both kinds of apps and download them.

---

3 *Moment* – Less phone. More life. https://inthemoment.io/
*Checky* Phone Habit Tracker on the App Store - iTunes - Apple. https://itunes.apple.com/us/app/checky-phone-habit-tracker/id912482478?mt=8

2. Write in your own words what this verse means to you: "Do not be afraid, little flock, for your Father has been pleased to give you the kingdom" (Luke 12:32 NIV). Do you believe it? Why? Why not?

3. To whom do you address your prayers—God, Jesus, or the Holy Spirit? When and why?

4. Spend a moment acknowledging God for who He is. Has He offered you grace, forgiveness, compassion, friends, funds, health, etc.? Let God's caring provision for you empower you today.

5. Think about a time when you needed a lap to curl up in or a shoulder to cry on, when you felt unloved, uncared for, or misunderstood. Tell Jesus about it. Idle down in prayer, calm your mind, and feel His comforting presence. Soak up His compassionate care. Feel His love encompassing you as you lose yourself in the peace He provides. Write about your experience.

## Chapter 6

# Tech-Pecked or God-Directed

In chapter 2, we looked at Dr. Larry Rosen's research linking the current anxiety epidemic with cell phone use. He recently completed a study where he asked 216 students to install an app on their phones that measured how often they unlocked the device and how many minutes they spent using it during the semester. The typical student unlocked his or her phone more than sixty times a day, for a total of 220 minutes. That's nearly a staggering four hours of time a day on their phones—and that doesn't count laptops, tablets, or other electronic devices. That means that even when they are supposed to be studying, they are unlocking their phones three to four times an hour to check in with social media and other electronic connections, and then they lock it back up again.

### FOMO

Rosen states, "People routinely check their phone every fifteen minutes, or less, often without an alert or notification. If we take their phones away, they get highly anxious until it is back in their possession." Not only does Rosen conclude that our performance is compromised by our smartphone obsession, our anxiety levels are increased as we suffer from FOMO: "Fear Of Missing Out."

Rosen states that "FOMO isn't actually a fear as much as it looks like a form of 'technological anxiety' that continues to rise until we check in with whatever is making us feel that way, and will abate only to start to rise again and again."

He suggests that we glance at our phones for different reasons. We may go on Facebook or other social media sites to view a cute cat video and share it with a friend. When we do, we smile. But there are also times when we feel relief from FOMO—a fear that we have not missed out on something that someone has posted, or that our friends are doing something fun without us. The fear of not being in the know about some important news break, or who's hosting a fabulous party, or even where a trending food truck will be parked that evening, compels many digital users to check their devices far more than is necessary or prudent. It's not as much about finding fun as it is about not missing out on something that might be epic. Living tech-pecked is generating epidemic anxiety in us.

These responses represent two different processes in our brains. According to Dr. Rosen, when we are compelled to engage in an activity to gain a feeling of pleasure, that behavior is connected to addiction. If, however, we participate in an activity and feel a sense of relief that we didn't miss out on something, this most likely is a sign of obsession. Addiction and obsession—we need to pay attention.

Rosen submits, "If I had to estimate the contributions to our behavior, I would say that our data support about a 3:1 ratio of anxiety reduction to pleasure." While our tech obsessions foster anxiety, that is the opposite of what life in Christ offers.[1]

Learning to spend time idling down in God's presence brings peace. Take a look at the contract He offers—and we don't have to pay more for an upgrade to get it. Psalm 29:11, "The LORD gives strength to his people; the LORD blesses his people with peace" (NIV). Isaiah calls Jesus "the Prince of Peace." And Jesus Himself makes this statement in John 14:27: "Peace I leave with you; my peace I give you. I do not give as the world gives. Do not let your hearts be troubled and do not be afraid" (NIV). Peter, who had his troubles as a

---

1 Larry Rosen, "This Is The Real Reason You Can't Stop Checking Your Phone," *Psychology Today*, July 14, 2015; https://www.psychologytoday.com/blog/rewired-the-psychology-technology/201507/is-the-real-reason-you-cant-stop-checking-your-phone

Christ-follower, wrote this about the Lord when he figured things out: "Casting all your anxiety on Him because he cares for you" (1 Peter 5:7 NASB).

## Tools to Live God-Directed Lives

So, let's look at this logically. We can live tech-wrecked, feeling constantly anxiety-ridden about missing out on we-don't-know-what. Or we can live God-directed, managing our digital distractions and quieting our hearts to feel peace in the Lord's presence. What sounds best to you? Isaiah shares God promise in Isaiah 26:3: "You will keep in perfect peace all who trust in you, whose thoughts are fixed on you" (NLT). We can't keep our thoughts fixed on God if we are interrupted six times every hour, and if we are on our phones for four hours a day surfing the net or trying to manufacture a connection with virtual friends. We have a choice to clear our heads and calm our minds.

Maybe the idea of spending time talking to God is hard for you to wrap your head around. But it's real; it's a game changer; and here is what it looks like. Make an appointment with God as the first thing you do in the morning. The truth is that we can meet Him any time of day, but without the opportunity to dose up on the strength He provides, you just might find that the day proves to be too much for you. Jesus set the example for getting up early to spend time with His heavenly Father, so if it worked for the Savior of the world, it's a good example to follow.

Set up a place to meet with God, like your favorite recliner, the patio chair on your deck, your kitchen table, or whatever works for you. Put everything you plan to use in this special place. Then you won't spend half an hour looking for your Bible, or your glasses, or where you left your journal. And you can avoid starting your day in frustration by wasting valuable time that could be spent quieting your soul and hearing from the Lord. Keep your phone facedown unless someone is on a road trip and you know that their car is acting up, or a loved one is currently in a life-threatening surgery. Do you see how specific this is? We can easily make excuses for keeping our phones on for any number of unnecessary reasons. But spending time getting our tanks full in the company of the Creator of the universe trumps looking at pictures of your friend's tailgate party or even checking out your cousin's latest Pinterest pin.

Get a good devotional. Anything by Sarah Young will work. Sarah writes as though Jesus is speaking directly to the reader. In fact, here is a quote from her book *Jesus Calling* about spending quality time with the Lord: "Come away with me for a while. The world, with its nonstop demands, can be put on hold. Most people put Me on hold, rationalizing that someday they will find time to focus on me. But the longer they push Me into the background of their lives, the harder it is for them to find Me."[2] There is so much truth in these words, and they provide compelling motivation to meet with God.

Open up your devotional and let it guide you into the presence of your waiting Lord. So often when I (Beverly) sit down to spend quiet time, allowing God to calm my mind, a thousand details, and at least two thousand worries, along with three thousand things on my to-do list, threaten to rob me of that time to refresh. It helps me to set a pad and a pen by my Bible and write down those things I fear that I will forget—in my case, I know I will forget. But I stay with my connection time with God. With all of that swirling around in my mind, it would be so easy to get up and get busy. I conclude that it's too hard to focus, so I should just give up. But I can't because this time is too valuable.

Don't let Satan rob you. We have this incredible privilege of spending quality time with Jesus and letting the light of His presence illuminate our path. It doesn't get any better.

David understood it. He writes in Psalm 32:8: "I will instruct you and teach you in the way you should go; I will counsel you with my loving eye on you" (NIV). And again in Psalm 16:11: "You make known to me the path of life; you will fill me with joy in your presence, with eternal pleasures at your right hand" (NIV).

If you're still not convinced of the benefit of spending time to let God lead you, then listen to the words of Jesus Himself: "I am

2 Young, op.cit., 208.

the vine; you are the branches. If you remain in me and I in you, you will bear much fruit; apart from me you can do nothing. If you do not remain in me, you are like a branch that is thrown away and withers; such branches are picked up, thrown into the fire and burned. If you remain in me and my words remain in you, ask whatever you wish, and it will be done for you. This is to my Father's glory, that you bear much fruit, showing yourselves to be my disciples" (John 15:5–8 NIV).

If we don't remain, we can likely crash and burn. The word *remain* in the Greek means "to continue, to tarry, to abide."[3] And the more we abide in His presence, the more He resides in our hearts and our heads to guide us and assure us of His undeniable love. Jesus continued, in John 15:9–11: "As the Father has loved me, so have I loved you. Now remain in my love. If you keep my commands, you will remain in my love, just as I have kept my Father's commands and remain in his love. I have told you this so that my joy may be in you and that your joy may be complete" (NIV). We can feel that joy as we continue, as we tarry in His presence. We open up His Word to read His love letter to us, and we talk to Him in prayer as we listen for His gentle whisper to guide us.

To look more at what it means to abide in Christ's presence, let visit again our steps to an A+ connection with God. In the previous two chapters, we examined the first two steps—Ask and Acknowledge. We can ask God for what we want and need. C. S. Lewis writes, "We must lay before Him what is in us, not what ought to be in us."[4] While it might seem more spiritual to pray for other people who are hurting rather than focusing on our own needs, prayer is about relationship. It's about "getting real" with our friend, and Jesus is the Friend who knows all about us anyway. So, we might as well let Him know what is on our hearts. He appreciates our honesty more than any false piety that we might try to muster.

---

3 James Strong, LL.D, S.T.D., *The New Strong's Exhaustive Concordance of the Bible* (Nashville, Thomas Nelson Publishers, 1910), *see remain.*
4 C.S. Lewis, *Letters to Malcolm: Chiefly on Prayer* (New York: Harcourt, 1992), 35.

As we ask Him for what we want and need, we are acknowledging His power to provide for us. That brings us to our next **A: Align**—we align ourselves with God's will for us. We can discover that plan for us collectively as we read about it in His Word. We uncover His plan for us individually as we talk to Him, as we listen to Him in prayer.

While there is discipline in prayer, desire motivates us more than duty. That is why we don't worry about our words. We talk to Him freely about who we are. We share openly about what we want in life, just like we do with our best friends, knowing that He is the Best Friend we could ever have. The more time we spend in prayer, the more we realize His unconditional, unquenchable love. That motivates us to spend even more time in His presence, but building faith takes time. In the last two chapters, we examined two of our **3 A's**: For an A+ Connection with God: **Ask**, and **Acknowledge**. Now let's explore the last **A: Align**, and what it means to align with God's plan for us.

## Align

Sometimes we align ourselves with God's plan more out of default than by making a deliberate decision, but He proves Himself faithful in spite of our doubts. When Bev and I gave our hearts to the Lord in that little country church on that hot and sticky summer Sunday in Tennessee, we knew we wanted to do something for the Lord after all He had done for us. The more we talked about it, the more we realized that we were on the same page with our dreams and aspirations.

Soon after that we each received a brochure in the mail entitled "Student Tips from Azusa Pacific College." It seemed too good to be true: a place that was devoted to teaching people about God, and it was in California to boot! We thought surely that students must surf between classes; we didn't realize that Azusa was fifty miles inland! The truth was that Azusa, California, seemed as far as away as we could get from the craziness and dysfunction of our home life, and that's where we wanted to be.

We prayed every night that God would make that happen, although we had no idea how we were going to get from Tennessee to California. We applied ourselves to our studies, becoming straight A students, and we dared to dream of a life away from anger and abuse.

One night when Mama wasn't in her usual irritable mood, Bev and I approached her about the idea. So much for her not being in an irritable mood! Our fears that she wouldn't like the idea were correct. Mama constantly reminded us that since the day my dad had left, she'd had to work, and so we had to work, and that's what we did. We took care of the cooking, dishes, laundry, cleaning, and babysitting of my little brother. It was clear that she was determined to keep us in that role forever.

When we finally got into bed that night, Bev commented, "Mama's not about to give up her cheap labor that easily." She was right, so we prayed all the more.

We would go to church and ask the youth group to pray with us. Youth group was our lifeline. Richard, the youth pastor, would listen to all of our questions about God and faith. He patiently answered every one of them, never making us feel dumb or like a bother.

Then one evening he walked into youth group with a heavy heart. "I need to let you all know that I'm going to be leaving. Anna May, the kids, and I are relocating to Memphis. We'll be moving in two weeks."

We were devastated. What would we do without Richard? He was the reason we came to church. He was our instructor, counselor, and encourager in our newfound faith. The day Richard moved away was one of life's saddest days to that point, and we had endured some pretty sad days. We couldn't even speak about it, our hearts were so burdened.

Within two months, Reverend Miller, the deep-voiced, kind-faced preacher who had welcomed us with a smile into sanctuary each week, announced that he was leaving the church as well. Tears welled up in his eyes as he told the congregation of his plans.

Church wasn't the same after that. The place we had come to for help, hope, and safety now seemed hollow and empty. We would have given up on God altogether if it wasn't for the words of the apostle Peter. When Jesus asked the disciples if they were going to desert Him like the masses had, it was Peter who responded, "Where else would we go? Who else has the words of life?" (see John 6:68). So we mustered the gumption to align ourselves in obedience to the Lord even though the folks who drew us to the faith weren't there with the encouragement we had come to crave.

Then one Sunday in the middle of our junior year of high school, as we sat in the morning service, a tall, slender man with the perfect timbre in his speaking voice stood up behind the pulpit. "My name is Everett Ashton. I am a graduate of Azusa Pacific College."

He clearly said many other things that day, but that was all we heard! Bev and I looked at each other and did our best to contain our excitement until the church service was over. Then we beelined to his office, flew through the door, and began talking at the same time.

After he was able to calm us down, he smiled kindly and said, "Don't worry, girls. The folks here at church have already told me all about your dedication to the Lord and your desire to go to a Christian college."

"They have?" I questioned, not realizing that anyone would be that thoughtful.

"I know the president of the college personally," Reverend Ashton continued. "I'll see to it that you get in."

We were speechless and shocked that a perfect stranger would show us such kindness.

A few short months later, Mama had a major "mother meltdown" and threw my sister and me out. We called our dad and he came to get us. One minute we were living in Chattanooga, Tennessee, getting ready to graduate from high school with honors, and the next minute we were in Charlotte, North Carolina, with a dad we barely knew, a stepmom we had met only once, and a little sister we didn't know existed. "This can't be good. Charlotte, North Carolina, is even farther away from California. Now we can really kiss our dream good-bye," I thought.

But Daddy was different from my mom. He cared about what his girls wanted.

"Ya'll are smart," he commented at the dinner table not long after we moved in. "You need to do something with all of your good grades. Where do you want to go to school? We have great schools around here, like Duke or Vanderbilt," he offered.

That was our cue. We poured out our hearts, again both talking at once, about our desire to go to a Christian college. State schools were practically free. That made it an even harder sell. But my dad loved us enough to support our dream. He had no money, but he helped us fill out the paperwork. I didn't see how it could possibly work out. Our friends were already getting scholarships, and it was easy to lose hope.

Six weeks after we sent off our applications, a letter arrived with Azusa Pacific College in the return address. I (Linda) handed the letter to Bev because I was too nervous to be trusted with the letter opener. The letter was from Cornelius Haggard, the president of the college. It read:

> I talked with Everett Ashton and he told me all about your de-
> sire to get a quality Christian education and how hard you have
> worked toward your goal. I want you to know that you are just the
> kind of young people we are looking for at Azusa Pacific. You are
> not only accepted but, with grants and scholarships, your way is
> completely paid. The last $1000 was supplied by a personal friend
> of mine from Hawaii—$500 for each of you. He, too, was moved
> by your story and determination. Welcome to California. We'll see
> you in the fall.

God honored our meager attempts to align with His will by blessing us despite our doubts and fears. Partnering with God requires faith. His miraculous provision builds our faith that He will continue to take care of us.

It was hard enough spending quality time getting to know God before the age of digital demands. Without quality quiet moments, it's difficult to grasp the depths of what relationship with God can do for us, especially when we are constantly bombarded with information overload. More and more researchers are jumping on the bandwagon encouraging us to manage interruptions, so that we can not only connect with those right in front of us, but so that we can think more deeply and creatively. In the next chapter we will explore what they are saying, and how we can idle down to find our deeper selves as we explore our connection with God.

## Making It Real

1. Do you have FOMO, the Fear Of Missing Out? Do you find yourself checking your phone to make sure that your friends or acquaintances aren't having fun without you? How do you feel when you check social media and realize that you actually have missed out on something?

2. Try one week of taking that tech-pecked time and devoting it to the Lord instead of your digital devices. Spend some time acknowledging God for who He is. Recognize His mighty power to create the world you live in and the beauty around you. Recognize all He has done for you and how He has led you on your life's path. Does that strengthen your faith and empower your prayer?

3. Take an inventory of your desires and see how they align with what you know to be God's will for you. Pray for courage to make the necessary changes to follow His plan for you. Ask someone you trust to help you be accountable for these changes.

4. Ask yourself—have you given up praying out of fear He won't give you what you want? Journal your feelings and let God know what is going on in your heart. Would you be willing to pursue the Lord, and let Him reveal His will to you? Journal what happens on your trust walk.

Chapter 7

# Disconnect to Reconnect

The demand that our digital devices have on our time is quickly surpassing the time we spend with the face-to-face real-live relationships right in front of us. The act of using a smartphone while in the company of someone in a social setting has become so prevalent that we as a society now have a name for it. We call it "phubbing," basically "phone snubbing." It describes when someone checks their phone while they are with others, ignoring them in favor of their smartphone.[1] When did we lose the art of talking without having to post selfies of our outings, or pics of our food, or worse, responding to our phone's every ping, ding, or buzz as we miss out on the opportunity to embrace real-live face time with those we care about? Living tech-pecked keeps us from tuning in to real people in real time. How many times do you walk into a restaurant to see entire families sliding into a booth with all of their faces engrossed in their phones and no one looks up to connect with anyone else? When did the post of a "friend" we barely know become more important that what is on our spouse's heart? When did the latest trending news article take precedence over finding out what our kids are being exposed to at school? It isn't just those close to us that our tech-pecked lifestyle keeps us from connecting

---

1 Orianna Fielding, *Turn Off Your Phone! Reconnect With Life* (England: Future Publishing Limited, 2018) 71.

with. We can be so digitally directed that we sacrifice valuable time connecting with our deeper selves.

## The Creative Process

You have probably heard of the Google effect. In 2011, psychologist Betsy Sparrow and her colleagues from the University of Colombia presented the first study on the "Google effect," with research showing how digital technology affects our memories. Their studies revealed that because we know that information is just a click away on the devices we carry around with us, we are less likely to try to remember information. Powerful search engines do the remembering for us. We no longer have to strain our brains to remember the facts we learned in school, or the name of the astronaut that was on the tip of our tongue. We let Siri do it for us.[2]

We can wonder, "What's the big deal? I don't need to clutter up my brain with trivia anyway, especially if my fingers can find it faster." However, memories are composed of complex, connected neurons that are strengthened every time we use them. Each memory is a bit of information encoded in the intricate piece of machinery we call our brains.

Sharon Begley, the senior science writer with *STAT*, a national health and medicine publication, writes, "New ideas come from novel combinations of disparate ideas, seemingly unrelated elements. Just as having many kinds of Legos lets you build more imaginative structures, the more elements—facts—knocking around in your brain, the more possible combinations there are, and the more chances for a creative idea or invention. Off-loading more and more knowledge to the Internet therefore threatens the very foundations of creativity."[3] In order to move into a state of flow that is needed for the creative process, our brains need uninterrupted periods of time, something that is in short supply in the Internet age.

2 Tyger, Latham, "Is Our Reliance on the Internet Making Us Dumber?" *Psychology Today,* July 16, 2011: https://www.psychologytoday.com/us/blog/therapy-matters/201107/the-google-effect

3 Sharon Begley, "Begley: Does the Internet Change How We Think?" *Newsweek*, January 7, 2010: https://www.newsweek.com/begley-does-internet-change-how-we-think-71085

## Three Days to a Richer Life

Some authors recommend taking time away from technology and spending quality time in nature to unplug and decompress. *New York Times* technology journalist Matt Ritchel accompanied several scientists, all of whom were studying the brain, on a retreat to a remote location in Utah. They decided to spend a week with no cell phones, no Internet access, and no digital distractions. The scientists wanted to observe what happened to their brains as they took a break from their digital devices in order to note whether it warranted further study for the rest of us in this wired-up world.

After three days of no tech, all of the scientists on the retreat noticed something significant happening. "You start to feel more relaxed. Maybe you sleep a little better. Maybe you don't reach for your phone pinging in your pocket," Richtel says. "Maybe you wait a little longer before answering a question. Maybe you don't feel in a rush to do anything—our sense of urgency fades." And research shows that along with that, your anxiety decreases.

One scientist attending the weeklong getaway observed, "I am not as engaged in my world when I'm constantly using devices as I am when I am away from them." Richtel terms this newfound feeling of freedom the "three-day effect." And the scientists concluded that this three-day effect could be the basis for future study that might help us understand what happens to our brains when we're overwhelmed with data, and what happens to us when we get away from it.

Weighing in on this concern, Matt Richtel concludes, "One way of looking at all of this research is to think of technology the way we think about food. Just as food nourishes us and we need it for life, so too—in the twenty-first century and the modern age—we need technology. You cannot survive without the communication tools; the productivity tools are essential. And yet, food has pros and cons to it. We know that some food is Twinkies and some food is Brussels sprouts. And we know that if we overeat, it causes problems. Similarly, after twenty years of glorifying technology as if all computers were good and all use of it was good, science is beginning to embrace the idea that some technology is Twinkies and some technology is Brussels sprouts."[4]

The truth, by anyone standards, is that whether we are ingesting Brussels sprouts or Twinkies, too much of anything can be a problem. Finding a balance leads to a healthier life. Just like the scientists concluded that monitoring their use of technology gave them more opportunity to tune in to the world right in front of them, the rest of us could find benefit from doing the same.

Disconnecting from our digital devices for periods of time each day may seem unnecessary and unwanted at best, and impossible at worst. But what if we told you that if you limited your brain's interruptions long enough to quiet your mind in prayer, you could not only greatly impact your own destiny, but you could influence the world.

## Prayer Makes a Difference to God

Throughout this book, we have continually built a case that the Creator of the universe, the One who set the stars in place, the God who spun the planets in their orbit, desires a relationship with you—the person sitting in your seat. The easiest way to respond to His offer of relationship is through prayer. But if you're like me (Linda), what you pray can be confusing.

For years I thought that God already had everything figured out, so it didn't really matter what we prayed, just that we prayed. Of course, my short-sided thought process didn't leave much room for Jesus' powerful request for us to ask, seek, and knock (see Matthew 7:7). But I stayed open, and I got my answer to this conundrum when I opened my Bible to Daniel 10. That's when I learned that our prayers make a difference to God.

While God knows everything, that doesn't mean He determines everything. He allows us the privilege of partnership with Him. That is a sobering thought, but we can see that as we read what happened

4 Heard on Fresh Air, "Digital Overload: Your Brain on Gadgets", *NPR*, August 2, 2010:http://www.npr.org/templates/story/story.php?storyId=129384107

to Daniel the prophet in this passage. When I first came across this section in the Old Testament, I felt like I had stumbled onto one of faith's significant insights. Grabbing additional reference books and commentaries for clarity, I discovered that my newfound truth had already been well researched. That only added to its value.

The scene opens with Daniel the prophet awaiting a message from God for His people. He was fasting and praying expectantly for God to reveal His vision. As he prayed, Daniel received a vision. Daniel 10:4–6 tells us: "On the twenty-fourth day of the first month, as I was standing on the bank of the great river, the Tigris, I looked up and there before me was a man dressed in linen, with a belt of gold from Uphaz around his waist. His body was like topaz, his face like lightning, his eyes like flaming torches, his arms and legs like the gleam of burnished bronze, and his voice like the sound of a multitude" (NIV). Topaz is a gemstone made of yellowish or brown well-formed crystals, brightly colored and shiny. You can imagine what Daniel must have felt seeing a vision like this![5]

The folks who were with Daniel didn't see the vision, but they were overtaken with fear and they fled and hid. That left Daniel alone, the only one left to see the formidable being. In Daniel 10:8 we read, "So I was left alone, gazing at this great vision; I had no strength left, my face turned deathly pale and I was helpless" (NIV).

Daniel 10:10–14 continues: "A hand touched me and set me trembling on my hands and knees. He said, 'Daniel, you who are highly esteemed, consider carefully the words I am about to speak to you, and stand up, for I have now been sent to you.' And when he said this to me, I stood up trembling. Then he continued, 'Do not be afraid, Daniel. Since the first day that you set your mind to gain understanding and to humble yourself before your God, your words were heard, and I have come in response to them. But the prince of the Persian kingdom resisted me twenty-one days. Then Michael, one of the chief princes, came to help me, because I was detained there with the king of Persia. Now I have come to explain

---

5 Merrill F. Unger, Unger's Bible Commentary on the Old Testament (Chattanooga: AMG, 2003), 1674.

to you what will happen to your people in the future, for the vision concerns a time yet to come'" (NIV).

*Unger's Commentary on the Old Testament* explains this prince as a demon exercising influence over the Persian realm.[6] Some theologians see this as Satan himself. The Prince of Darkness was waging war to keep God's message from reaching His people through Daniel. The being with the bronze body and the blazing eyes reported to Daniel that he had heard the prophet's prayer and had set out to give him the message he had been seeking. Then he adds, "But the prince of the Persian kingdom resisted me twenty-one days. Then Michael, one of the chief princes, came to help me, because I was detained there with the king of Persia" (Daniel 10:13 NIV). The *Holman Illustrated Bible Dictionary* explains that Michael is the angel who serves as the guardian of God's people.[7]

As the messenger made his way to Daniel, we see that he was detained by the powers of hell itself. For twenty-one days the impressive messenger along with Michael fought the resistance of demonic forces before he was able to deliver his divine message. While Daniel prayed, the battle raged, until the angel, with Michael's help, was able to fight through the resistance and deliver God's vision. Daniel had been fasting and praying for that twenty-one days. Daniel's prayers made a difference!

Let's look again at Daniel 10:12, where the angel gives credit to the fasting prophet: "Do not be afraid, Daniel. Since the first day that you set your mind to gain understanding and to humble yourself before your God, your words were heard, and I have come in response to them" (NIV). The angel is conveying that from the moment Daniel started to pray, his words were heard, but Satan tried to prevent the prophecy from getting to him. Still, his faithful prayers and his perseverance moved the hands of heaven on behalf of him and his people. His prayers made a difference to God!

What a lesson! So much for my thinking that God had everyone's life dialed in and the universe neatly determined. This story

---

6 Unger, ibid.
7 Chad Owen Brand, Charles W. Draper, Archie W. England, *Holman Illustrated Bible Dictionary* (Nashville, Holman Reference, 2003) 1119.

in Scripture showed me that my prayers make a difference to God. Then I came upon this quote by C.S. Lewis that further validated my thinking. With brilliant insight into the dilemma of whether we should even bother to pray because God already knows what is going to happen, C.S. Lewis offers this illumination: "The event has been decided—in a sense it was decided before all worlds began. But one of the things taken into account in deciding it and therefore one of the things that really cause it to happen, may be the very prayer that we are offering."[8] That information changed my passion for prayer. I now pray, knowing that the words I am offering up may be woven into the fabric of the very answer that I seek. I feel both the responsibility and the privilege of being part of God's miracles.

## Prayer Makes a Difference in Us

Not only does prayer make a difference to God, but prayer also makes a difference in us. In Daniel 10:15–19, we read, "While he was saying this to me, I bowed with my face toward the ground and was speechless. Then one who looked like a man touched my lips, and I opened my mouth and began to speak. I said to the one standing before me, 'I am overcome with anguish because of the vision, my lord, and I am helpless. How can I, your servant, talk with you, my lord? My strength is gone and I can hardly breathe.' Again the one who looked like a man touched me and gave me strength. 'Do not be afraid, O man highly esteemed,' he said. 'Peace! Be strong now; be strong.' When he spoke to me, I was strengthened and said, 'Speak, my lord, since you have given me strength.'"

The "one who looked like a man" was the preincarnate Jesus Christ, who touched Daniel and gave him strength to replace his fear. It was that same Jesus Christ who showed up for Elijah as he sat under the broom tree despondent and discouraged because Jezebel was trying to kill him. He brought Elijah water in a drought, food in a desert, and hope in the midst of his fear (see 1 Kings 19:1-18). When we call on the Lord, He personally answers us and gives us the comfort and hope we need. Prayer makes a difference to us.

8 C. S. Lewis, *Miracles* (New York: McMillan, 1947) 187.

## Daddy's Light

When we need the Lord, He is there. He was there for our father when Daddy needed Him most. Cancer was sucking the life out of this once-vibrant, delightfully funny man. He battled valiantly for five years, but he was failing quickly. I (Linda) lived on the opposite end of the continent, so it was hard for me to travel back to see him. But when the doctors recommended hospice care, Bev called me to let me know that I needed to come right away while he still knew that I cared enough to be there.

When I arrived it was obvious that our stepmother, Barb, was exhausted from caring for him. So, when our younger sister, Renee, came into town, she and I (Linda) convinced Barb to take a day and rest. "The two of us can handle Daddy's care while you go home and sleep for a while. Otherwise we'll be taking care of you," Renee informed her.

After Barb painstakingly helped her husband of forty years to a chair, she agreed to take us up on our offer.

Daddy sat up for a while, but it was obvious he was in a lot of pain. Just before lunch he wanted to lie down. Renee and I walked him across the room to his bed. After fluffing pillows and rearranging covers until we felt that he was as comfortable as we could possibly make him, we headed toward the couches at the far side of the hospice room to catch up while Daddy slept.

Renee didn't hear him, but I did. Clutching his covers until his knuckles were white with pain, he whispered, "I hate this."

I walked back to my father's bedside. I took his hand and said, "Daddy, I'm so sorry you hurt. I'm so sorry you are in this pain." Then I did what my faith had taught me to do when I didn't know what to do. I prayed aloud, "Lord, You know Your son is hurting, and You promised that we could come to You, and that You would give us rest. Let him rest in Your arms of peace right now."

Fervently lost in prayer, I was overcome by a permeating sense of peace. Then I felt a gentle tap on my shoulder. "Lin, look." It was Renee. She was standing on the other side of Daddy's bed, holding his other hand. As I opened my eyes, I saw a brilliant ray of light radiating between us and resting gently on my dad. His brow, which had been furrowed from the pain, was now relaxed. He slept serenely, enveloped in the glow. The light still shining, Renee began to pray out loud for my dad. When she finished, I started again. I don't know how long we remained in that sacred moment.

We were interrupted by a knock at the door. It was a longtime family friend who had come by to check on my dad. I ushered him to the sitting area of the hospice room so that my dad could sleep while we talked.

Our visitor didn't stay long, and the minute he walked out the door, Renee jumped up and said, "Could you believe that light? I'm so glad you were here, Lin, because no one would believe me. I'm not sure I would believe myself!"

"I'm glad you're here too," I agreed.

Just then Renee's husband, Bill, joined us. She rushed to tell him our story. From the way he rolled his eyes, I could tell he wasn't buying a bit of it. Bill is a wonderful Christian man who makes his living as an airplane pilot, but he was not about to be taken in by the emotion of the moment.

Turning on his heels, he walked over to the window next to the bed where my dad lay sleeping. He returned to the sitting area wide-eyed and slack-jawed.

"Ya'll, there's a building in front of that window," Bill reported, shaking his head.

"I know," I explained to my skeptical brother-in-law. "You can't say it was just the sun shining through the window and explain this away as some natural occurrence."

Bill seemed to soberly let this soak in.

My stepmom returned from a day of much-needed rest accompanied by Bev. We left Bill to watch my dad, and we crossed the hall to the kitchen, where wonderful church folks from all over town brought in meals for the hospice families each week. We ate quickly in case my dad woke up and needed something, but as we did, Renee recounted the story about our prayer and the light. "This radiance was bright yellow," she offered. "And glowing."

"It enveloped the room," I chimed in.

We both struggled for an adequate description, as we stated at the same time, "It had substance."

Though my father didn't come to Christ until later in his life, Christ came to him in that hospice room in the presence of a radiant light to bring him rest and comfort, and to bring those of us present His peace.

God has made us for connection with Him. We can find that life-giving connection when we take the time to disconnect from the immediate and move to the deeper places in our hearts and souls, when we invest in what is eternal. We've learned that prayer moves the hands of God—it makes a difference to Him. When we connect with Him, it generates a difference in us as we pray. And as with my dad, it makes a difference in the person being prayed for, even when they are unaware. Now we get to look at what prayer shows us about God Himself—that He isn't different. He isn't like us, subject to different moods. He is trustworthy, and He can be counted on, as we see in the next chapter.

## Making It Real

1. Are you a "phubber"? What does it cause you to miss out on? What can you do to change that?

2. Try to disconnect from your tech for three days. See if the "three-day effect" is real to you.

3. Set a goal to turn off your technology while you are spending time in prayer. If you receive your daily devotionals from an app on your phone and that creates too much temptation to get busy online, opt for a hardbound devotional instead.

4. How do you feel when you read how Daniel's prayer moved the hand of God? Does this inspire you to be more persistent in your prayer life? Write out a prayer for someone or something that you have practically given up on. Let it serve as a reminder to persist in prayer for your answer.

5. Reflect on this C.S. Lewis quote: "The event has been de-cided—in a sense it was decided before all worlds began. But one of the things taken into account in deciding it and therefore one of the things that really cause it to happen, may be the very prayer that we are offering." What do you feel impressed to pray for right now? Lift those prayers to the Lord, knowing your participation is part of His divine plan. Write out your prayers.

6. How has the Lord graciously answered your prayers as He did by bringing comfort and sleep to our dad?

7. Write down any unmistakable answers to prayer that you have received from God through prayer. If you have not yet experienced an unmistakable answer to your prayers, ask God to reveal Himself to you and keep your eyes open ev-ery day to look for His involvement in all of your moments.

# Chapter 8

# I-Life or Real Life

Experiencing God's peace in a transforming way takes intentionality, and it takes time. But we can be so wired up to outside stimuli from Facebook, Twitter, Instagram, Snapchat, and all
the others that we are too preoccupied to find God in the midst of
our moments. Yet our frenetic pace creates a need for His peace all
the more.

I (Beverly) recently read a story about a band of nomads in Africa who would stop along the path in their travels "for their souls
to catch up." At first, my enlightened mind took pity on these unin-
formed travelers. Then I joined the ranks of the media generation,
and I found myself longing to slow down since my body seemed to
constantly outrun my weary soul. My judgmental attitude now gives
way to envy as I admire my wise brothers and sisters who take the
time to rest, and I constantly pursue a quiet place to turn down the
noise in my mind.

Our relentless attachment to our phones keeps us tech-pecked
and prevents us from taking time to connect with the feelings,
thoughts, and insights that we can find in the deeper places in our
souls, because our minds are bombarded with images and ideas,
with data and decisions, on a constant basis.

## 15-Minute Tech Breaks

Dr. Larry Rosen wrote an article for the March/April edition of *Healthy Living Made Simple* magazine in which he states: "We have this device that we love, that contains everything we could ever want—information, connection, our pictures, our music—but that is also driving us nuts and making us anxious about our world." Rosen suggests that we take tech breaks, and he offers an example. "During certain times of the day, set your alarm for fifteen minutes and put your phone upside down on your desk. When the alarm goes off, give yourself one minute to check in. Then reset your alarm for another fifteen minutes. Just keep doing this until it feels comfortable."

Rosen also recommends that after taking a tech break, talk with your family about how it felt. "Did you feel anxious? Did you feel free? Did your kids notice, 'Hey, Mommy and Daddy paid more attention to us?' Did your spouse enjoy watching TV together or lying on the bed and talking instead of being on devices?" He closes by offering, "This helps raise awareness and motivation."[1]

Limiting the digital domination in our days is a step on the path to finding inner peace. But there is more we can do to move from tech-pecked to tuned in as we seek to find God in a world addicted to noise and speed. Here are 3Rs that can restore peace and reconnect you with yourself and God: **Reflect, Release, and Rest.** Turn your phone off and spend some time soaking up the benefit of time with the lover of your soul.

## Reflect

In Psalm 46:10, we read these instructions: "Be still and know that I am God" (NIV). It's hard to stay focused in this fast-paced culture, but we grow weary in the rat race, and who wants to be a rat anyway? That's when this verse brings the insight we need. The word for "still" in the Hebrew is the word *raphah*. It means "to slacken, to cease; to be faint, feeble, or idle; to leave alone or let go; to draw toward evening." If you're Southern, it's like you're sitting on

1 Larry Rosen, Ph.D, "Being Smart About Screen Time," *Healthy Living Made Simple*, (March/April 2018) 16-17.

your front porch swing sipping sweet tea waiting for the lightning bugs to show up.

This word implies that we surrender our agenda, and that can be hard to do. We have places to go and people to tweet! Yet unless we can simmer down, we will miss something powerful, because the root word for *raphah* in the Hebrew is the word *rapha*, which means "to mend by stitching, to make or cause to heal or repair, to thoroughly make whole."[2] The Lord is telling us to calm down, to quiet our minds so that He can thoroughly heal us. He wants to give us His peace over our pieces, but if we are not present in the moment, we will miss this gift.

The book of Psalms has more to teach us about the peace that God provides. In Psalm 16:11, the psalmist David extols, "You have made known to me the path of life; you fill me with joy in your presence, and eternal pleasures at your right hand" (NIV). Again, in Psalm 21:6, he reiterates, "Surely you have granted him unending blessings and made him glad with the joy of your presence" (NIV). David spent a lot of time seeking God. We see that as he makes his point once more in Psalm 89:15–16: "Blessed are those who have learned to acclaim you, who walk in the light of your presence, O LORD" (NIV). In the New American Standard Version the word for "presence" here is "countenance."

## God's Countenance/Disposition Toward You

In the Psalms, David continues to speak poetically about seeking God's face, or countenance, and spending time in His presence, and we wonder if this is just colorful language or if there is really something to the idea of actually seeking the face of God, or the light of His presence. What would that look like if we could achieve it?

Let's dig deeper for more understanding. The definition offered for *countenance* in the *Encarta Dictionary* is "somebody's face, or the expression on it." When used as a verb, it means "to tolerate, accept or give approval to something."[3]

2 James Strong, LL.D, S.T.D., *The New Strong's Exhaustive Concordance of the Bible* (Nashville, Thomas Nelson Publishers, 1910), *see still.*
3 Microsoft Encarta Multimedia Encyclopedia, Microsoft Corporation (1993-2009),

79

In the original language, *countenance* included both the noun and the verb. One's face is an indication of mood, emotion, or character. As we focus on the Lord's countenance, we idle down and focus on His disposition toward us. One's disposition is an inclination or tendency to act in a particular way.[4]

God reveals His disposition toward His people in His Word: He has good things for you. He values you, and He wants to take care of you. This verse proves it: "Now that we know what we have—Jesus, this great High Priest with ready access to God—let's not let it slip through our fingers. We don't have a priest who is out of touch with our reality. He's been through weakness and testing, experienced it all—all but the sin. So let's walk right up to him and get what he is so ready to give. Take the mercy, accept the help" (Hebrews 4:14–16 MSG).

Jeremiah 29:11 reads, "For I know the plans that I have for you, declares the LORD, plans for welfare and not for calamity to give you a future and a hope" (NASB). Perhaps you have experienced your share of calamity in your life, and like us, you have watched God prove Himself again and again in spite of fearful circumstances.

When we limit competing distractions, take our eyes off the fear we're facing, and focus on the face of Jesus, we can soak up the peace He provides, along with the deep sense of well-being that everything will be okay. The more we feel the Lord calm our fears and clear our heads, the more we become convinced that He is a good God who can be trusted.

## The Light the Lord Provides

That is what Natalie experienced. As a young mom with three active boys all under the age of six, she found little time to be still. When her husband announced he was going to be laid off, she knew she had to make that time.

"We had just worked out our finances so I could quit my teaching job, and I was so enjoying being home with the boys. I was

*see countenance.*
4 Hollman Illustrated Bible Dictionary, (Nashville, B&H Publishing, 2003), *see countenance.*

commuting an hour one way, and they complained a lot about how they never saw me.

"I kept thinking, 'Does this mean I have to go back to work? We just got this house. Now will we have to give it up?' I tried not to dissolve into tears," she candidly shared.

"I told myself, 'I can fall apart when I am alone.' So, I breathed a prayer for strength to get through the rest of the evening and plowed ahead.

"I made a nice dinner for my husband that night. I could tell he was feeling defeated, even though I know he was trying to stay as positive as possible. I figured making him his favorite meal would lift his spirits.

"After cooking, cleaning up, bath time, and wrestling the boys to bed, I sat down, turned off my phone, and opened up my Bible. I needed some insight, some inspiration to break through the fog of fear, confusion, and weariness in my mind. As I sat quietly, I felt the urge to look up the word *light* in the concordance in the back of my Bible. I know now that was the 'still, small voice' of God speaking to me and guiding me along."

The first reference for *light* that Natalie found was in John 8:12: "When Jesus spoke again to the people, he said, 'I am the light of the world. Whoever follows me will never walk in the darkness, but will have the light of life.'" That led her to Luke 1:79 as she read Zechariah's prophecy concerning the work of Christ, "to shine on those living in darkness and the shadow of death, to guide our feet into the way of peace." The fog was clearing as the tears were forming, when she read the next promise in Psalm 31:14–16: "But I trust in you, LORD; I say, 'You are my God. My times are in your hands.... Let your face shine on your servant; save me in your unfailing love.'"

"Those words wrapped around me like a warm quilt," Natalie shared. "I lifted my head to dry my eyes and caught a glimpse from my living room window. The full moon shone behind the snow-capped mountains and enveloped them in a golden glow, and all the while I felt enveloped in a quiet peace in the light of God's presence.

What resonated in my head in that moment was that I could hold my problems lightly in light of God's presence."

"That peace followed me for days to come. Before, I had felt like a battery that had been nearly discharged with all the stress I was feeling, and those quiet moments alone with the Lord and His Word restored the 'charge' I needed to keep me in that peaceful state. I found that as I continued to wait for an answer to my prayers, I couldn't hold on to that peace without spending quiet moments 'being still' in the Lord's presence. I had to return to that peaceful place, focusing on the light of the Lord to recharge my spiritual battery," Natalie confided with a smile.

God wants us to gaze into His face, so that He can change ours. Reflecting on God's amazing capability gave Natalie the ability to release her worries to Him and trust in His competent care. That brings us to the next *R* that brings restoration to our stressed-out souls.

## Release

Mark was a hardworking husband and a dedicated father. He managed to attend church here and there, but it never mattered much to him until his younger brother dropped dead of a heart attack at forty-eight. Suddenly all things spiritual greatly mattered in his life.

"My brother was into God and really involved in his church. It blew me away that his seventeen-year-old son, Jason, stood up in front of everyone at his dad's funeral to tell us how much he respected his father. Jason said his dad had led the boy's campouts for church each year and taught him and his friends about God. My young nephew shared with all of his dad's friends that he knew he would see his father again someday," Mark shared.

"That made me realize that something was missing in my parenting. If anything happened to me, I would want my son to be confident and strong like that." I (Linda) could hear both grief and newfound conviction as Mark opened up.

"My mom and dad took us to church when we were young. I went until I moved out on my own. That's when I sowed my wild oats and prayed for a crop failure, as the saying goes." We both laughed to lighten the mood for the moment.

"I'm not proud of the choices I made during that time. There are things that if people knew, they wouldn't let me in the church doors." He paused, looking at me for a response.

"Mark, I'm not nearly as worried as you are about the roof caving in if you show up at church, because I know who God is, and He's never stopped loving you despite what you may think. He's looking for guys just like you." He smiled, as I continued. "My old pastor used to say, 'If you don't feel close to God, guess who moved?' Many times we don't go to the Lord because we are not convinced we are worth His while. We feel too messed up to even ask for His help. And that's the very reason Jesus died for us. But when we can own our bad and let it go, we can move past it. We just need to confess it to God, and be free of it!"

"You make it sound so simple. I've been pretty convinced that God would not be happy with the likes of me."

"You don't have to take my word for it, Mark. You can trust the Lord. He's been reaching out to you for a quite a while. What do you think got you here?

"I have some homework for you," I continued. "Sit down with a couple of hours stretched out ahead of you, put your pen to the page, and write down everything you feel bad about, every dastardly deed. Don't hold back. If you want to be purged of the pain, you gotta do the work.

"Then pray and ask God to forgive you of your sin, and believe that He will. After that, it's important that you ceremonially destroy the paper. Throw it into a fireplace, shove it down a paper shredder, or tear it into tiny little bits and dump it into a nearby lake, but do something memorable so that you have a reference point for your moment of forgiveness. When Satan uses guilt to throw your sin in your face, you can remind him, and yourself, that your sin has been forgiven, and you can recall the moment in time to prove it.

"Do you remember having a chalkboard in your classroom as a kid?" I figured he was about my age so he could relate to my example.

He nodded.

"When I was a kid, the teacher would erase what was written on the board every day. But once a month or so, she would bring in a bucket of water and a sponge to clean the large green chalkboard that stretched from one end of the classroom to the other. As she wiped her wet sponge across the board removing any traces of old writing and even the finest chalk dust, the green board popped with color and clarity. As the Lord's forgiveness wipes our hearts clean from the fine chalk dust of sin and guilt, we can experience cleanliness and clarity that truly sets us free."

"I'm ready," Mark declared.

"So is God," I assured him.

Sometimes the struggles that keep us from connecting with God aren't as clear to us as Mark experienced. He recognized that he continued to recycle his guilt because he didn't feel worthy of God's forgiveness. Once he knew what he had to do, it was a matter of doing it. When he was able to release himself to the Lord, he found the freedom his soul craved, and a sustaining relationship with a Higher Power he could lean on.

## Counseling Sessions with God

But what if you find yourself stuck? Your thoughts are unsettling, and it's difficult to pinpoint the cause. You would like to release your burdens to the Lord, but you need more clarity to know what those burdens are, to understand the exact nature of what's troubling you.

I (Linda) have stumbled onto a tool that has been very helpful when I get stuck. I have named this tool my **Counseling Sessions with God**, and here's why. As a pastoral counselor for the past thirty years, I have a lot of experience with how counseling sessions flow. The client comes in, shares his/or her presenting issue, talks for a while, then expects the counselor to reflect back on what was said and offer clarity regarding the issues that were laid out.

With this pattern in mind, I idle down in my Divine Counselor's office, under a tree, beside a rock, in my office, anywhere in the universe will do since He owns it all. But before I can remotely hope to hear from God, I have to silence the tech-pecked voices from every digital portal, and that is no easy feat. Before all of the research that precipitated the passion to write this book, FOMO compelled me to rivet my face to my tech connections. Opening my computer to check my email invited me to view the latest news. While I was there, an ad would show up for the magic potion lotion that was going to melt off my body fat with only three easy payments. They even took PayPal! With my computer opened, I might as well see how my one thousand friends were doing on Facebook, and if my phone buzzed, any hope of pensive deep thought was quickly terminated. Please understand that my husband and I pastor a church of over a thousand people. That is a lot of people in need. But if I allow my schedule to be dictated by constant digital overload, I will have no time with God to fill my tank to help with their needs. Not picking up the phone is a sacrifice, but it is well worth it to preserve my own sanity and to give me time with God to better equip me for action when I do make contact. I learned that the hard way.

With my digital devices disconnected, I pick up pen and paper (I know, so old school, right?), and I write out what is consuming my thoughts. My mind can run a thousand miles a minute, but as I simmer down, I can get in touch with the deeper layers of what I'm thinking and feeling. If I am seriously troubled, I simply start with what I am feeling right now in this moment, just as a client would do in my office. Writing is better than talking because it slows me down and fine-tunes my focus. As I write, I ask the Lord to speak into my life.

I write until the issue crystallizes. Sometimes that happens in a few lines. Other times it takes a few pages. But I find as I slow down enough to write, I can better hear the Lord's "gentle whisper."

## God Speaks

A pastor friend of mine explains that God often speaks to us as "an interruption of thought." As I quiet myself, my mental commotion dies down, and a crystal-clear thought often dispels all the others. When God is trying to get my attention, it's not just some random interruption. It's a clear, succinct thought that provides peace and offers help. The wisdom and clarity presented are far beyond my ability to conjure up in that moment, leaving me more convinced than ever that the message is divinely inspired.

As that clarity comes, I write down those words just as I have written my thoughts and feelings, but I'll highlight the current words of wisdom. I may need to keep writing to finish getting my feelings out, but I can come back later to those words of insight for the answers that I am seeking. Then I read and reread the counsel they offer me.

Please understand, I am not one of those people who claim, "I do whatever the voices in my head tell me to do!" The interruption of thought I am referencing here is uncluttered by confusion and unencumbered by fear, and it possesses a power to bring peace and an assurance that it is the Truth. The old saints of the Church would often call that one's "Inner Witness" referring to the voice of God in each of us who follows Him, or the presence of the Holy Spirit seeking to guide us from within.

## The Inner Witness

The Inner Witness, God's gentle whisper, or a divine interruption of thought are all ways we seek to wrap words around what defies explanation, God speaking to us. It is something more easily experienced than explained, but we can always check the validity of the message by God's Word. He won't contradict Himself. So, the crazy-eyed guy on TV who says that God told him to kill a certain person clearly didn't hear from God!

God can't go against His nature, and that nature is represented in the person of Christ, who, as He walked the earth, loved sinners, encouraged saints, and died to prove it. Even if my counsel that day from the Lord is corrective, it never comes from a place of anger or disgust. It's helpful and uplifting for me and for the people in my life.

My counseling sessions with God have supplied me with answers as straightforward as, "Let go of your offense. That person doesn't mean to hurt you," to as specific as, "Now is not a good time to make major purchases." Sometimes it's a reminder of what I already know—that God has a plan, and that He can be trusted to take care of my problems no matter how difficult they seem in the moment.

All this goes without saying that if I am at the end of a cell phone leash, I won't be able to quiet my heart long enough to commune with my Creator. Like the tribe of nomads mentioned at the beginning of this chapter who stop during their travels for their souls to catch up, our souls can catch up with our busy minds when we employ the **3Rs for Restoration: Reflect, Release,** and **Rest,** with the last one being the hardest.

Would you believe that there are people who have to work at resting? Maybe you are one of them. I (Beverly) know that I am one. The very meaning of the name *Beverly* is "Industrious One," and I have spent most of my life living up (or down) to the meaning, depending on your perspective. Technology only fueled my busyness. I once set a New Year's resolution to be lazy! Like most of my resolutions, I had failed by mid-January. I now call myself a recovering over-doer. In our next chapter, we will look at what it means to unplug in a culture that's plugged in 24/7.

### Making It Real

1. Try the "family tech break" that Dr. Rosen suggested at the beginning of this chapter. Encourage everyone in the house to disconnect from tech for an hour or two together. Following up with a discussion time is a must.

2. In the discussion time, consider how being unplugged made each family member feel. Be prepared for pushback. Tech addiction is real. Be persistent to help your kids move toward healthier habits and be ready to hear that they like you better without a phone in your face.

3. Reread the section in this chapter about God's countenance— His disposition toward you. Remember, one's disposition is an inclination or tendency to act in a particular way. What do you assume to be God's disposition toward you?

4. Read these verses to influence your response.

   - Jeremiah 29:11
   - Isaiah 41:10
   - Jeremiah 31:3
   - Zephaniah 3:17
   - Psalm 37:23–25

From what you have read, write two to three sentences that declare how God feels about you.

5. Reread the verses that Natalie read: John 8:12; Luke 1:79; Psalm 31:14–16. Have you ever experienced peace in a storm like Natalie in this chapter? Write about it.
6. Ask yourself if you have let your past sins set you back as you struggle to believe that you are fully forgiven. Perhaps you need to complete the exercise prescribed for Mark in this chapter and release your load of guilt as you walk into the light of truth. Make that happen—now.
7. Carve out some time to unplug. Leave your devices behind, and with an old-fashioned pen and paper, plan a counseling session with God. You might not have a pressing issue to write about, but time spent listening for His voice will provide you with immeasurable peace and power.

Chapter 9

# Unplugged—Rest for Your Mind, Body, and Soul

All too often our constant online connection can become an obsession. Then we can't turn down the noise in our heads long enough to rest, much less to hear from God.

When our faces are pasted to our screens late into the evening, we're not restoring our bodies with much-needed sleep. While more and more studies are confirming the importance of sleep for our mental and physical well-being, equally as many studies are warning us that our sleep is being robbed by late nights with blue lights.

In a study posted in the *Harvard Health Letter* entitled "Blue Light Has a Dark Side," researchers revealed that exposure to light at night throws the body's circadian rhythm off balance. Your circadian rhythm is basically a twenty-four-hour internal clock that is running in the background of your brain and cycles between sleepiness and alertness at regular intervals. It's also known as your sleep/wake cycle.

Light suppresses the secretion of melatonin, a hormone that influences circadian rhythms. While light of any kind can suppress the secretion of melatonin, blue light at night does so more powerfully. Harvard researchers and their colleagues conducted an experiment comparing the effects of 6.5 hours of exposure to blue light to exposure to green light of comparable brightness. The blue light suppressed melatonin for about twice as long as the green light and shifted circadian rhythms by twice as much (3 hours versus 1.5 hours).

Research continues to link lower melatonin levels with more problems than just sleeplessness. In a Harvard study, researchers put ten people on a schedule that gradually shifted the timing of their circadian rhythms. Their blood sugar levels increased, throwing them into a prediabetic state, and levels of leptin, a hormone that leaves people feeling full after a meal, went down.[1] The study shed light—no pun intended—on the link between light at night and obesity and diabetes. Living tech-pecked robs us of our health.

## The Dangers of Tech for Kids

In an article for *Healthy Living Made Simple,* Dr. Jeffrey Bernstein warned parents of the allure of electronic devices. As kids stay up late indulging in life online, depression and anxiety increase because of the interruption of sleep cycles that we mentioned earlier. The noted psychologist states, "Not surprisingly, a lot of exhausted kids who feel very depressed start to feel anxious because they are worn down, and kids who are anxious start to feel depressed, creating a vicious cycle."[2] They aren't the only ones getting caught up in this consuming cycle. As adults, we miss the rest that our bodies and souls need as we overindulge in the information age. Yet, as we resist constant immediate involvement, we can idle down to the deeper places in our souls and find the rest and peace that God provides. That can be easier said than done.

## Rest

Resting from technology—resting at all—is becoming so foreign in today's wired-up world that we decided to make a thorough scriptural study of what it means to take a rest. First, let's look at a working definition of the word as a starting point.

---

1 Harvard Health Letter, "Blue Light Has a Dark Side" *Harvard Health Publishing,* August 13, 2018, https://www.health.harvard.edu/staying-healthy/blue-light-has-a-dark-side
2 Jeffrey Bernstein, Ph.D, "Anxiety and Depression: Not Just For Adults," *Healthy Living Made Simple,* (March/April 2018) :12-13.

The *Encarta* dictionary defines *rest* as: "(noun) state or period of refreshing freedom from exertion or a rhythmic pause between musical notes. (Verb) to be in a state of tranquility or to cease activity."[3] In Scripture, there are several words used in the Old Testament for *rest*.

In Psalm 116:7 we read, "Return to your rest, my soul, for the LORD has been good to you" (NIV). In order to gain the full impact of what David is saying, we should start at the beginning of that chapter.

In Psalm 116:1–9, David writes, "'I love the LORD, for he heard my voice; he heard my cry for mercy. Because he turned his ear to me, I will call on him as long as I live. The cords of death entangled me, the anguish of the grave came over me; I was overcome by distress and sorrow. Then I called on the name of the LORD: 'LORD, save me!' The LORD is gracious and righteous; our God is full of compassion. The LORD protects the unwary; when I was brought low, he saved me" (NIV).

After all of this David extols, "Return to your rest, my soul, for the LORD has been good to you. For you, LORD, have delivered me from death, my eyes from tears, my feet from stumbling, that I may walk before the Lord in the land of the living" (Psalm 116:7–8 NIV).

The word for "rest" in this verse is the Hebrew word *mnuwchah*, pronounced men-oo-khaw`.[4] I (Linda) always hate to see a word written out, especially in another language, without a hint of how to pronounce it. Pronunciation turned out to be important to Bev and me when we became Southern transplants to a California college. Our newfound friends continually encouraged us: "You've gotta talk faster if you expect anyone here to listen." They were right. For both of us at the time, "no" was a three-syllable word. But I digress. (Now my friends say that my spiritual gift is making a short story long!)

Back to *mnuwchah*. The word in the Hebrew is what we think of when we read the *Encarta* definition for "rest." It means to repose peacefully, to be comfortable, at ease, quiet, or still. Because of God's complete care, we can relax and rest regardless of our circumstances. That flies in the face of the addiction to activity in the age in which we live.

---

3 Microsoft Encarta Multimedia Encyclopedia, op. cit., see rest.
4 Strong, op. cit., see *rest*.

Sitting quietly in the Lord's presence is a discipline we can learn. We won't find the deep peace that God provides rushing through our days. As we turn down the noise in our minds and press into His presence, we will find peace in the midst of pain, calm even in chaos, and triumph over any trial. Just like Natalie did in our last chapter.

## Fired from Running Your Own World

The prophet Isaiah uses a different word as he instructs his readers in Isaiah 30:15: "This is what the Sovereign LORD, the Holy One of Israel, says: 'In repentance and rest is your salvation, in quietness and trust is your strength'" (NIV). The word for "rest" used in this verse is the Hebrew word *nachath*, pronounced *nakh`-ath*. (Sounds a bit like Klingon, doesn't it?) It means "to sink, to descend, to come down, to depose." The definition for "depose" is "to remove someone from office or position of power."[5]

As a kid in church, I often heard my youth pastor ask, "Who is on the throne of your life? Is it you, or are you letting the Lord reign in your desires and decisions?"

Yet another word is used for *rest* in Psalm 37:7: "Rest in the LORD and wait patiently for Him" (NASB). Before I give you the literal meaning of this word for *rest*, it would be helpful to check out the psalmist's message leading up to his instructions to rest and wait for the Lord.

## Soft and Pliable

David writes in Psalm 37:4–6, "Delight yourself in the LORD; and He will give you the desires of your heart. Commit your way to the LORD, trust also in Him, and He will do it. He will bring forth your righteousness as the light and your judgment as the noonday" (NASB). To really get the full value of this section, we have to not only explore the word *rest* in the original language, but we need to dig deeper into the meaning of the word *delight*.

Usually, to delight in someone or something means to take great joy or pleasure in that person or thing. That is one of the meanings

5 Ibid.

for *delight* in the Old Testament, but that is not the word for *delight* that David chose to use in Psalm 37:4: "Delight yourself in the LORD and he will give you the desires of your heart." The word for *delight* here means "to be soft and pliable to the will and purposes of God. And He will bring you salvation, satisfaction, plan, and a purpose— the very thing your heart desires."[6] The longer we follow Jesus, the more we become like Him, and the more easily our desires fall in line with His desires for us.

When I (Beverly) came to faith as a kid, I thought that if I agreed to follow the Lord, He would call me to some far-off jungle in Africa, where I would have to live in a hut with a dirt floor and where the indigenous people would want me to eat monkey meat! Now, after all these years of following the Lord, I am pretty convinced that if the Lord wanted me to go to Africa, then that is where I would be the most happy and fulfilled. God's faithfulness in my life, time and time again, has made it easier to trust Him when I find it hard to understand what is happening and why. The more I trust Him, the easier it is to be soft and pliable to His will and His ways.

The more we surrender our agenda to the Lord, the more fulfilled we become. The more we dare to trust the Lord, the more He proves Himself trustworthy. Then we find He either gives us what we desire or transforms our hearts to desire what He gives us. As we seek to be soft and pliable to the Lord's leading, and as we commit our way to Him, we find that He will bring forth our righteousness as the light and our judgment as the noonday, as promised in Psalm 37:8.

David goes on to add, "Rest in the LORD and wait patiently for Him" (NASB). Now we can investigate what the word *rest* means in this passage. The Hebrew word is *damam*, pronounced *daw-mam`*, and it means "to be dumb, (implied) to be astonished, to stop, hold peace, quiet self, put to silence."[7] When we remain teachable before the Lord, we seek to die daily to our own selfish desires and we embrace God's desires for us. As we submit ourselves to the Lord and let Him mold us to His will for us, we will find ourselves astonished

---

6 Ibid, see *delight*.
7 Strongs op.cit.,see *rest*.

at His mighty work in our lives. His miracles, peace, and provision can leave us speechless in awe and gratitude.

It is not always easy to rest like Isaiah 30:15 teaches by pulling ourselves off the throne of our lives and letting God have that rightful place. Nor does it come naturally to remain soft and pliable before the Lord like Psalm 37 instructs, but God helps me when I ask Him. Paul tells us in Philippians that God will not only help us do what He has called us to do, but He will even give us the "want to"—the desire to do His will. Philippians 2:13 states, "For it is God who works in you to will and to act in order to fulfill his good purpose" (NIV).

In his series *Not a Fan*, Kyle Idleman teaches that when it comes to living a godly life, it's not about trying daily; it's about dying daily.[8] When we die to selfish choices or to our right to be irritated, angry, proud, or jealous, and we let the Holy Spirit live through us, we will be glazed, dazed, and amazed at the strength and peace that He provides.

It's all but impossible to discover soul-strengthening revelation when we can't find rest. And it's just as impossible to find rest when our trigger fingers never leave our devices. If we want to go to the deeper places in our souls and in our faith, it takes time. That may mean restricting time that we spend currently indulging our obsession to check the latest email or explore what's new on Facebook. Constantly keeping up with the latest bit of news and gossip, whether it's from our friends or MSN, can be exhausting, but our FOMO can make us slaves to our devices.

In the next chapter, we will explore currently trending ideas about meditation to help us unplug from the constant bombardment of digital information that comes at us at lightning speed 24/7. We will examine tools to help us unwind, followed up with scriptural support that can move us from reactive to relaxed, from frenetic to finding peace in the presence of the living God.

---

8 Kyle Idleman, *Not a Fan: Follower's Journal* (Louisville, City on a Hill Studio, LLC., 2010)105.

## Making It Real

1. Try refraining from looking at a screen for two hours before bedtime. Record your sleeping cycles for the next two weeks to see if it makes a difference.

2. Which Old Testament word for *rest* resonates the most with you and why? Psalm 116:7: to repose peacefully, to be comfortable, at ease, quiet, or still. Isaiah 30:14: to rest from running your own universe. Psalm 37:8: to be so astonished you are totally quiet and can't even speak. Write down your thoughts about each verse.

3. In Psalm 37:4 we read, "Delight yourself in the LORD and he will give you the desires of your heart" (NIV). It would be easy to look at this verse at face value and insist that God should give us what we want because we are "delighting" in Him by being believers. How does it change the meaning of the verse when the correct word from the Hebrew is presented—which means to "be soft and pliable" before the Lord? Write about what this means to you. How hard is it to follow these instructions and why?

4. What does Idleman's phrase, "It's not about trying daily; it's about dying daily," mean to you, and how can you appropriate that in your life?

5. Make an honest appraisal of why you check in with tech. Be open to learning more about setting boundaries with your digital devices as you keep reading.

Chapter 10

# Mindful Meditation
# Isn't Just for Monks

As often happens with twins, Bev and I, on opposite ends of the continent and without ever conferring with each other, began to study the topic of meditation at the same time. As a couple of type-A personalities with demanding jobs that require connection to many people both digitally and face-to-face, we found great benefit from the tools we discovered, and which we would now like to share with you.

With the increase in digital overload, anxiety has hit an all-time high, and so has our interest in meditation. Is it possible that constantly being linked up has created a driving need in us to wind down? For decades, Christians have stayed away from meditation for fear that it was a New Age practice or rooted in something that was not of God. However, meditation is as old as the writing of the Psalms, and more and more information is coming to light that Christian meditation, when done properly, can be healing for the brain as well as the mind, body, and soul.

Meditation conjures up the idea of listening to sitar music as you sit cross-legged on the floor while endlessly chanting the same word over and over again. That's not exactly the idea that modern meditators present. Making its way to newsstands and blogs everywhere is *mindful meditation*. In the past, it's been utilized and promoted in Buddhist practices, causing many Christians to stay away from it lest they get sucked into false teachings. But we know that even with its new explosion in current culture, David in the Old Testament spoke about the benefits of meditating long before Buddha ever came on the scene.

It's important as Christ followers not to get swept away by the plethora of the secular information about meditation, or anything else for that matter, and the best place to go to prevent that is Scripture. So we heed Paul's words in Colossians 2:8: "See to it that no one takes you captive through hollow and deceptive philosophy, which depends on human tradition and the elemental spiritual forces of this world, rather than on Christ" (NIV). Our goal is to let Scripture dictate how we form our philosophies for living.

Here is what the Word tells us about David's commitment to meditate on the Lord and His teachings. He states in Psalm 119:48: "And I meditate on your decrees" (NIV); in Psalm 119: 27, "Cause me to understand your precepts, that I may meditate on your wonderful deeds" (NIV); in Psalm 119:78,"But I will meditate on your precepts" (NIV); and in Psalm 119:148, "That I may meditate on your promises" (NIV). *Meditation* is mentioned twenty times in the Bible, and eighteen of those references are in the Psalms alone. Because David spoke of meditating on some aspect of God constantly in his writing, it is easy to wonder if that is how he survived the challenges of being a warrior king who was constantly on the run from people he loved.

John Baker, the founder of Celebrate Recovery, writes, "Prayer is talking to God. Meditation is listening to God on a daily basis. When I meditate, I don't get into some yoga-type position or murmur, 'om, om, om.' I simply focus on and think about God or a certain Scripture verse or maybe even just one or two words."[1]

Joshua 1:8–9 states: "Keep this Book of the Law always on your lips; meditate on it day and night, so that you may be careful to do everything written in it. Then you will be prosperous and successful. Have I not commanded you? Be strong and courageous. Do not be afraid; do not be discouraged, for the LORD YOUR GOD will be with you wherever you go" (NIV).

1 John Baker, *Celebrate Recovery Leader' Guide,* (Grand Rapids, Zondervan,1998) 196.

In a world without digital bombardment, David and Joshua had longer stretches of time to ponder the deeper places of their souls and the love of the Lord. For us, living in a world in which we are constantly connected up to information overload, calming our hearts in the presence of our Lord and Savior can prove to be one of our greatest challenges.

Cognitive therapists have employed the relaxation tools used in mindful meditation along with therapeutic self-talk to help clients reduce stress and anxiety, with great results. In his book *I Want to Change My Life*, Dr. Steven M. Melemis coupled mindful meditation deep-breathing exercises with positive thinking and created what he called "Mind-Body Relaxation."[2] Focusing on positive self-talk is certainly effective for life change, but focusing on God's Word brings His power to us in the process. Utilizing the relaxation techniques borrowed from mindful meditation and proven effective in cognitive therapy, we've created a template that helps the user soak in God's Word to create life change. We call it **Let-Go-and-Let-God Meditation.** Here are the steps; we will break each one of them down for you.

- **Breathing:** While breathing focus on either your nostrils or your abdomen to help you shut out every distraction and pay attention to the Lord.
- **Relaxation**: Allow your body to relax and follow along.
- **Thought Surrender**: Surrender each thought to the Lord.
- **Be Present**: Stay in the moment.
- **No Judgment**: Suspend judgment of yourself, others, and your circumstances, and accept the present moment just as it is.
- **Gratitude:** Spend some time in God's presence thanking Him for all He has done for you.

If you've spent any time in church, you have been taught the benefit of having a quiet time with the Lord. While I (Linda) dedi-

2 Steven M. Melemis, Ph.D. M.D, I Want To Change My Life: How To Overcome Anxiety, Depression, and Addiction, (Toronto, Modern Therapies Ltd., 2010) 11.

cated time to be with God every day, I always had to compete with my crazy-busy mind. The constant pinging thoughts in my brain rob me of the moment. My active mind flits with thoughts, from alligators to xylophones and anything in between. My to-do list would often steal my focus and breed anxiety despite my best efforts to calm down and soak up the peace God offers. On the rare occasion when my racing mind could be still enough to experience the Lord's presence, my tank was filled to overflowing. But those moments were few and far between. My meditation practice now helps me turn down the noise in my head and quiet my anxious thoughts so that I can hear from God.

The first thing I do every morning is head to my desk, where I have a standing appointment with the Almighty every day. Actually the very first thing I do is stumble to the coffeepot to fill my cup—and *then* I head to my desk.

To create a quiet space, I have to silence my devices. I open my devotional book before I open my computer or turn on my phone because I know that if I don't, my focus will be carried away to everything from answering the latest email to jumping down a rabbit hole of updates about my friends and family. I love keeping up with people and reading the latest posts on my favorite blogs. I enjoy getting the latest world news and even catching up on the gossip from pop culture—and yes, I even love cat videos, but not if these things rob me of time with the God of the universe. I need the strength that being with God brings more than anything else in life. Perhaps you do, too. Here are some tools to help you employ the relaxation of mindful meditation as you idle down to spend quality time with the Creator of the universe. So, turn off your phone, leave your laptop closed, and open up to what God has for you.

## Tool 1 for Let-Go-and-Let-God Meditation: Breathing

Focus on your breathing, either at the nostrils or at the abdomen, to help you shut everything else out and pay attention to the Lord.

Breathing deeply oxygenates the brain, and that helps us to think more clearly. And, of course, it honors God when we set aside time specifically to seek Him. In Isaiah 26:3 we read, "You will keep in perfect peace, all who trust in you, all whose thoughts are fixed on you!" (NLT). As we soak up time in the presence of the living God, we can fix our thoughts on God as Isaiah instructs or we can fixate on our problems, those we care about, or our never-ending to-do list. Focusing on the former alleviates anxiety. Focusing on the latter only increases it.

Sarah Young, writing from Christ's perspective to the reader, shares: "When you approach me in stillness and trust, you are strengthened. You need a buffer zone of silence around you in order to focus on things that are unseen. Since I am invisible, you must let your senses dominate your thinking. The curse of this age is over-stimulation of the senses, which blocks out awareness of the unseen world."[3] Without the constant ping, ding, or buzz from an onslaught of worldwide information, we have more opportunity to idle down and hear from our Creator.

## Tool 2: Let-Go-and-Let-God Meditation: Relaxation

Allow your body to relax and your mind will follow along.

Have you ever experienced tense moments, when, no matter how much you tell your brain to relax and let go, your worries continue to dictate your mood? Neuroscience teaches us that the brain is wired for worry. It is Velcro for negative and Teflon for positive. A large function of the human brain, particularly the amygdala, is designed to keep us safe. It doesn't like unpredictability, so it tries to figure things out. When it cannot complete that task, repetitive ruminations can occur and get "stuck" there. The more we ruminate and worry, the more we habituate the brain to that practice, and it becomes our norm. So, worry begets worry.

That's why relaxing the body and mind is so helpful. When we focus on relaxing physically, then our mind takes the hint. Breathing deeply and rhythmically moves us toward a relaxed state. As we focus on our breathing, it moves our minds from our plans, irritations, or problems to what our body is doing. Because our

---

3 Young, *Jesus Calling*, op.cit., 174.

bodies exist in the present moment, when we focus on our breathing, we are in the now.

Lamentations 3:22–23 tells us, "Because of the LORD's great love we are not consumed, for his compassions never fail. They are new every morning; great is your faithfulness" (NIV). As we calm our bodies, our minds can stop racing long enough to comprehend the compassions that God makes available to us. So much captures our attention in our action-addicted world. We will miss His many blessings, His compassions, if we are too wired up to wind down long enough to listen for the gentle whisper. That quiet time in His presence, steeping ourselves in the peace He provides, is vital to our well-being. It's our spiritual lifeline.

When it comes to resting in God, we can become our own worst enemy and fight the very thing that helps us most. In *The Message* translation, Isaiah 30:15 reads, "God, the Master, The Holy of Israel, has this solemn counsel: 'Your salvation requires you to turn back to me and stop your silly efforts to save yourselves. Your strength will come from settling down in complete dependence on me. The very thing you've been unwilling to do.'" When we can relax in the Lord and stop trying to solve all of the problems and issues we're facing by ourselves, we are able to find God's peace over our pieces.

Focusing on our breathing helps to calm our spirits, relax our bodies, and quiet the noise in our heads. Meditation experts explain that a relaxed body is "grounded." Before we dismiss this as "crazy yoga-talk," let's look at this from a scientific perspective. When you're tense, your body doesn't rest comfortably. You're ready to fight or flee, and your muscles lift you up slightly to prepare you for what's ahead. You're figuratively on your toes. When you're relaxed, you rest firmly on the ground. Grounding yourself is simply feeling your body just where you are in the seat, in a room, on the street, on this planet that God created. Your body and your mind are present now, not worrying about the past or the future. Your brain is more malleable or changeable when you are in a grounded state. Breathing deeply helps you to become grounded.

Relax your face. Your face registers your body's tension. The easiest way to relax your face, believe it or not, is to smile. Almost as much of your brain is devoted to controlling the muscles in your face as is devoted to controlling the rest of your body.[4] Bringing a gentle smile to your lips relaxes muscles from your eyes down to your jaw; plus it helps you recognize what this exercise is all about—seeking joy in the presence of Jesus, even in the midst of stress.

## Tool 3 of the Let-Go-and-Let-God Meditation: Thought Surrender

**Surrender each thought to the Lord.**

When a thought, a worry, or even a plan comes into your mind, let it go and give it to God, because your purpose is to be in the now experiencing God's presence in the present. That's your present! This is such an important step that we have named this entire exercise the **Let-Go-and-Let-God Meditation.**

First Peter 5:7 tells us, "Cast all your anxiety on him because he cares for you" (NIV). The Greek word for *cast* here is less intentional or deliberate of an action than words used elsewhere in Scripture for *cast*. In comparison, in Mark 9:42, Jesus states, "If anyone causes one of these little ones—those who believe in me—to stumble, it would be better for them if a large millstone were hung around their neck and they were cast or thrown into the sea" (NIV). The word *cast* in Mark describes a more deliberate action. It means "to eject, to expel, to drive out, and to thrust away." In 1 Peter, the Greek word for *cast* that Peter used means to "fling with a quick toss." We are to fling away our troubles, our worries, our anxiety. We flick them away and give them to Him. A quick flick of the wrist, and we let each problem, care, or concern go. I (Linda) will even say as I pray, "That's Yours, God; that's Yours, God," as I let go of all the worries and cares that collect in my mind.

I figure it this way. I can fling or I can linger. I can cast my concerns on the Lord, or I can wrap up in the latest post about terrible

---

4 Melemis, op.cit., 52.

happenings across the globe, the mess in my head, the circumstances that aren't going the way I think they should, my problems, or the one's I've borrowed from tomorrow, or I can fling them onto Jesus and relax in the moment. Once I give the Lord my burdens, the hardest job becomes not to take them back onto myself. That's when I have to be consistent. As soon as I realize that I am fixating on my thoughts again, I give them back to Jesus. This goes on until, at last, even for a moment, I leave them there. I (Beverly) tell my clients that when a worrisome thought starts, they should take both hands and vigorously dust their shoulders off like they are flicking off an annoying bug. Then they should state the annoying thought out loud and fling it into the Lord's capable hands.

It's not always easy to let go and let God. Maybe you were raised in a family with the motto, "If it's going to be, it's up to me"? Being needy or even depending on anyone else was looked upon as weak. Perhaps the people you did depend on proved to be utterly untrustworthy. So, you made a plan, either consciously or subconsciously, to take care of "*moi*" because nobody else would. It's what you do. First Peter 5:7 is a difficult verse for the self-reliant because if we give it God, whatever it is, we're not in control of it anymore (like we ever were anyway). But as we look deeper at these words and their author, Peter, we gain more understanding.

Peter thought he had it wired. At the Last Supper, when the Lord was telling His disciples what was going down, Peter kept insisting that he would stand strong. He told the Lord in Matthew 26:35, "Even if I have to die with you, I will never disown you" (NIV). That very night, Peter's pride didn't hold up. He denied the Lord, and the rooster crowed.

Now read the words of the repentant Peter in his first epistle as he teaches, "Humble yourselves, therefore, under God's mighty hand, that he may exalt you up in the proper time. Cast all your anxiety upon him because he cares for you. Be alert and of sober mind. Your adversary, the devil, prowls about like a roaring lion, looking for someone to devour. Resist him, standing firm in the faith..." (1 Peter 5:6–9 NIV).

This is written for the self-sufficient, and Peter should know. Before we can cast our problems on the Lord, we first have to humbly realize that we can't do this life with its challenges, demands, and troubles on our own. We need to trust Someone who is far better qualified to handle them—Jesus. We cast them on Him because He cares for us. Peter goes on to warn us that Satan doesn't want us to trust the Lord. He wants to keep us wrapped up in our problems, trying to figure them out on our own and remaining miserable in the process. When we give our problems over to the Lord, we can rest in His ability to take care of whatever life dishes out and stand firm in our faith.

As we breathe deeply and offload our worries onto the Lord, who is far more capable of handling them than we are, we recognize that we can do our best, and trust the rest to the Best while we rest!

If you have a hard time letting go of your problems, offloading the thoughts that stress you out and threaten to trap you in your stinkin' thinkin', you aren't alone. And you aren't "doing it wrong" if that happens. It's the nature of our brains to wander, especially when we are stressed. But don't give up. The more we practice letting go of our thoughts and leaving them with Jesus, the easier it will become to actually leave them there.

## Tool 4: Let-Go-and-Let-God Meditation: Be Present Stay in the moment.

I (Beverly) struggle with staying in the moment. I'm a planner, and planners fall prey to control issues. They think that planning is a wise and good thing. But all good things have their downside, and planners tend to live in tomorrow not today. Last year my word for the year was "NOW." Wow, was it hard for me. But I realized that all of my planning and controlling took me away from the simple pleasures of being in the present—the warm breeze on my face, the twinkle in a two-year-old's eyes as he says, "Nana" for the first time, and especially feeling the presence and power of a loving Jesus who wants me to just be with Him.

Listen to the advice of Jesus Himself in Matthew 6:34: "Give your entire attention to what God is doing right now, and don't get worked up about what may or may not happen tomorrow. God will help you deal with whatever hard things come up when the time comes" (MSG). If we are convinced that God will give us what we need when we need it, we can concentrate on being in the now. It requires a conscious effort to push back the demands of time and intentionally rest in the moment we are in. There is always something that needs to be done, someone who needs to be contacted, some tidbit of information calling to us from the digital world of endless stimulation, but God is waiting to bless us with His peace in the now.

We stay in the moment by continuing to focus on what is happening with us physically as we breathe. Our bodies exist in the now, so when we focus on them, we connect with the moment. Then we can honestly pay attention to the thoughts that we are surrendering, and see that so many of them are thoughts of regret about the past, or worries and fears about the future. We worry about what is going to happen to people we love, or how we are going to get through the ever-mounting to-do list for today and the days ahead. We can waste a lifetime pining after the past or fretting about the future and never realize that life exists in the current moment.

Just as she did in *Jesus Calling*, Sarah Young shares in a first-person perspective in her book *Dear Jesus*, as if the Lord is speaking directly to the reader: "Instead of gazing into the unknown future, live each moment in joyful awareness of My Presence.... I alone have access to the 'not yet,' because My existence is not limited by time. As you go step by step through each day, I unroll the future to you. While you walk forward on the red carpet of time, you never set foot on anything but the present moment. Recognizing the futility of future-gazing can help set you free to live more fully in the present. The freer you become, the more you can enjoy the reality of My Presence."[5]

The present moment is where the Lord desires to truly bless us

5 Sarah Young, *Dear Jesus* (Nashville, Thomas Nelson, 2007) Young, 224-225.

with His presence. That is where the power is. We can't control the future, but if we saturate our souls with trust in the Lord and believe that He's got good things for us, we can relax and let Him do His job, while we live in the moment and enjoy what is right in front of us.

Along with awareness, mindfulness involves acceptance.

## Tool 5: Let-Go-and-Let-God Meditation: No Judgment

**Suspend judgment of yourself, others, and your circumstances, and accept the present moment just as it is.**

Don't even judge yourself because you are having trouble being present or because your mind tends to wander. Just let that go like a cloud floating away.

When we embrace the moment we're in, and recognize that it is all we have, a new acceptance of life as it is, not as we wish it was, or worry that it will be, emerges. This acceptance of life as it is, in the now and in the moment, precludes any harsh judgments of ourselves. As we quiet our hearts and rest in God's presence, we are more able to embrace what He thinks about us rather than nursing and rehearsing our own negative self-talk. We can let go of ruminating about regret, fretting about the future, and/or pining away about the past.

Sometimes as Christians, we can be our own worst critics. In an effort to "live a life worthy of the calling," we can become self-critical, full of doubt and self-loathing. Compound that with rejection and abandonment brought about by our family-of-origin issues and we have a recipe for self-judgment that doesn't improve our performance. It leaves us anxious and unhappy as we seek to perform to feel like we are lovable.

When I (Beverly) came to Christ, I believed that He forgave me because that was a result of His mercy and grace, but it was my performance that I doubted. If couldn't please a mother I could see, it was hard to believe that I could please a God that I could not see.

While I could never live up to my mother's expectations, as a cowering codependent I didn't stop trying. I became a performance junkie excelling in everything from academics to band. I became a leader in every club, and I auditioned for every play, along with keeping the house clean and doing dinner, dishes, and laundry every night. Despite my best efforts, the love and acceptance I desperately desired from my mother always seemed to escape me.

When I came to Christ, without even realizing it, I projected my fear of not being enough onto God. But the more I read in His Word, the more I realized His love was not based on my performance. The more time I spent reading His promises and talking to Him in prayer, the more I became assured that He loved me, warts and all. And that had nothing to do with my performance. Thank goodness!

Still, the tendency of living as a "human doing" rather than a human being has been a tough habit to break. I can be quite the "Accomplish-monster," wanting things to be different than they are and/or better because they can be. Remember, my name means "Industrious One." I can miss the moment by being consumed with what needs to be done, telling myself that I can relax just as soon as I can cross this next thing off my list or get this last problem fixed. All the while, the Lord gently invites me to stop fixing problems and fix my eyes on Him, my "ever-present help in trouble," as the psalmist writes in Psalm 46:1. He continues to teach me that He desires our presence, not our perfection. He wants our presence so that He can reassure our doubting hearts of His love and strength to help us.

We not only waste our time worrying about our own performance, but we can live in frustration about the behavior of others, and we can't control them. A simplified version of step one in twelve-step recovery states, "I admit that I am powerless over people, places, and things." I can fret my life away wishing and wanting other people to do or not do certain things, without recognizing how little power I have to affect that.

Acceptance does not imply resignation or giving up. We can pray for them and ask the Lord to work in us to bring them light, but we are not God's appointed Holy Spirit to "make them better." That's

His job. We have enough on our plates just staying sane ourselves.

Our quality time spent seeking the Lord bridges the gap between what is and how we want it to be. In the quiet of the present moment, absent of any judgment of ourselves, other people, or our circumstances, we can relax in God's presence and breathe out our problems as we breathe in God's peace.

## Tool 6: Let-Go-and-Let-God Meditation: Gratitude

**Spend some time in God's presence thanking Him for all He has done for you.**

While we did not see this tool as part of the mindful meditation exercises represented in the various books and websites we considered, our research has uncovered what a game-changer living in gratitude can be. So, we made it a part of our **Let-Go-and-Let-God Meditation.** We recommend that you write out a list of everything you have to be thankful for. Call it your "Blessed List," and read that list regularly, especially when things aren't going well. It's easy to forget that God is working things out when life isn't going the way we want it to. Remembering the good things God has given us reminds us that He is in charge and that He can be trusted, no matter how daunting the circumstances.

Over and again in Scripture we see the significance of thankfulness. In 1 Thessalonians 5:18, Paul instructs: "Give thanks in all circumstances; for this is God's will for you in Christ Jesus" (NIV). In Colossians 2:6–7, again he shares, "So then, just as you received Christ Jesus as Lord, continue to live your lives in him, rooted and built up in him, strengthened in the faith as you were taught, and overflowing with thankfulness" (NIV). And in Philippians 4:6, he writes: "Do not be anxious about anything, but in every situation, by prayer and petition, with thanksgiving, present your requests to God" (NIV).

Dr. Daniel Amen shares his research in a piece he calls "The Hateful Brain vs. the Grateful Brain." He participated in a project with psychologist Noelle Nelson. Dr. Nelson was working on a book called *The Power of Appreciation* and had her brain scanned twice. The first time she was scanned after thirty minutes of meditating on all the things she was thankful for in her life. After the "appreciation meditation," her brain scan presented a very healthy, high-functioning brain.

Then she was scanned several days later after focusing on the major fears in her life. One of her major worries was about her dog. She fretted about the dog getting sick. She feared she would have to miss work to care for him. That could cause her to lose her job. That spiraled into her losing her apartment because she had no job, leaving her with no money to treat the dog, and down she went, mentally circling the drain.

Dr. Amen scanned her brain after she mulled on these thoughts. Her frightened brain showed serious decreased activity in two parts of her brain. Her cerebellum had completely shut down. That part of the brain is involved in physical coordination, such as walking or playing sports. New research also suggests that the cerebellum is also involved in how quickly we integrate new information. According to Amen, "When a cerebellum is low in activity, people tend to be clumsier and less likely to think their way out of problems. They think and process information more slowly and get confused more easily.

"The other area that was affected was the temporal lobes, especially the left one. The temporal lobes are involved with mood, memory, and temper control. Problems in this part of the brain are associated with some forms of depression, but also dark thoughts, violence, and memory problems."

"In Noelle's scans, when she practiced gratitude, her temporal lobes were healthier. When she frightened herself with negative thinking, her temporal lobes became less active. Negative thought patterns change the brain in a negative way."

Dr. Amen ends this passage in his book by stating, "Practicing gratitude really helps you have a brain to be grateful for."[6] The good

---

6 Daniel G. Amen, Change Your Brain Change Your Body: Use Your Brain to Get and Keep the Body You Have Always Wanted (New York, Three Rivers Press, 2010) 227-9.

doctor proved with technology what the Bible has supported for millennia: Living in gratitude changes how we view the world, the Lord, and ourselves.

In this chapter, we focused on tools to help us idle down and connect with God in prayer—not always an easy accomplishment. C.S. Lewis wrote, "The prayer preceding all prayers is 'May it be the real I who speaks. May it be the real Thou that I speak to.'"[7] These words can inform us as we seek, in the next chapter, to clear out the clutter that keeps us from connecting with Christ.

## Making It Real

1. Turn off the tech and tune in to God. Do you find when you want to spend quiet time in the Lord's presence that you have to compete with your crazy-busy mind? Does your to-do list threaten to steal your peace despite your best efforts? Set aside time each day to practice this Let-Go-and-Let-God exercise.

2. Reread Tools 1–6 to bring you clarity and help you remember where to go next, so that your meditation time can have more uninterrupted flow.

3. Instead of your brain telling your body to relax, try relaxing your body to inform your mind to relax. Journal about how that feels.

4. Do you find when you try Tool 3 that as you cast your cares on the Lord, your cares just keep coming? Does it help you to not feel so alone as you learn that everyone struggles with this? Does it provide you with motivation to keep "flinging your cares" on the Lord because He cares for you? Do you believe that the more you practice, the easier it will be to actually cast your cares and leave them there? How long do you think that will take? Is it worth it?

5. Does Tool 4—"Suspend judgment of yourself, others, and your circumstances, and accept the present moment just

---

7 Lewis: op. cit., 81-82.

as it is"—make you feel as though you are giving up or that you are trusting God more? Does it provide comfort to know that you don't have to be perfect? Does it help you relax and seek God in the present moment? Write about that.

6. Do you suffer from being an "Accomplish-monster"? In your family of origin, did you have to earn love by your accomplishments and achievements? Explore the possibility that you could be projecting these same expectations onto God. Write about that.

7. Reread Tool 6 and take the time right now to write a copious and thorough Blessed List, including everything you have to be thankful for—everything personally about you and your environment. Don't leave anything unstated. Then read your list three times a day for the next three weeks and add to it as you observe more blessings. Note whether the practice makes a difference in your mood and your perspective.

# Chapter 11

# Conversing with the Universe or a Caring God

Communication with the Almighty can be a heady concept, and it is further complicated by the amount of time we spend communicating with everyone else through our digital devices. Sure, we have a worldwide reach, but as a therapist who deals daily with communication issues, I (Beverly) am seeing that all this "communication" isn't producing the connections our souls crave.

More and more people share the angst-filled feeling of "being together alone." In the YouTube video *Look Up*, which has clearly struck a nerve with the corporate conscience of culture with its current 61,319,699 views and counting, Gary Turk states, "I have 422 friends and yet I am lonely. I speak to all of them every day, but none of them really know me." He goes on to say, "Be there for your friends and they will be there for you. But no one will be there if a group text will do."[1] He even ends his piece by telling the viewer to turn off his video and go out to engage in life.

Jean Twenge, a psychology professor at San Diego State University who has written prolifically on young people and mental health, recently released a study that shows a link between the rise of the

---

1 Gary Turk, "Look Up," *garyturk.com*, April 25, 2014: https://www.youtube.com/watch?v=x-9StdvEHMmw

smartphone and growing rates of depression, suicide attempts, and suicide itself among teens: "The finding is based on data compiled by the Centers for Disease Control and Prevention in the US and teen-related surveys. It revealed that feelings of hopelessness and suicidal thoughts had gone up by twelve per cent between 2010 and 2015. Nearly half of the teens who said they spend five or more hours a day on a smartphone, laptop, or tablet said they had thought about, planned, or attempted suicide at least once—compared to twenty-eight percent of those who said they spend less than an hour a day on a device."[2] The more young people live tech-pecked, the more prone they are to suicide ideations.

We can all agree that the more time we spend investing in something, the more influence it has on us. But we also have to agree that a lot of what we are getting bombarded with is not all good. The subtle and not-so-subtle influence of this bombardment can lull even the most steadfast Christ-follower to get sucked into philosophies and ideas that do not line up with Scripture.

## Praying to the Universe

One concern we've seen in the counseling office is tech-addicted believers, people of faith, in today's postmodern culture, who are easily influenced by media to pray to the universe, their enlightened selves, or whatever movement that catches the fleeting fancy of trenders and tweeters. When this endeavor fails to yield the desired results, they consciously or unconsciously give up prayer and even God altogether.

However, if we embrace the Bible as our guidebook for life, it will dictate how and what ideas we allow ourselves to embrace. After living over a half century on this planet and using God's Word to counsel thousands of people collectively, experience has taught us that Scripture has guidelines that benefit those who choose to live by them.

The Bible teaches us that when we pray, we can talk to the living God, not a nebulous entity or a universe designed to cater to our

2 Donna Vickroy, "Technology Triggers Teen Depression," *The Star Online*, January 8, 2018: https://www.thestar.com.my/tech/tech-news/2018/01/08/technology-triggers-teen-depression/

every whim—a trend that continues to surface in today's postmodern media. In fact, the Scripture presents quite a different picture. Jesus Himself tells us to expect trouble. In John 16:33, He said, "I have told you these things, so that in me you may have peace. In this world you will have trouble. But take heart! I have overcome the world" (NIV). Yet because we live in the land of plenty, with freedom and opportunity without oppression and abundance all around us, it's easy for us to think that we are entitled to an easy life in which everything goes our way. Then we look on Facebook, or, as one high-profile pastor called it, "Fakebook," and we see how everyone else has such an awesome life, we think, "So should I!" Let's face it: If you are having a hard day yourself, scrolling through delightful, smiling people eating cake or celebrating a great life event can be discouraging, even if you know it's not the total story.

However, what did Jesus promise? Trouble—irritable babies, IRS audits, car accidents, bum knees, job loss, hair loss, cellulite, and the list goes on. And sometimes these trials, the very things designed to draw us to God, are the things our entitlement causes us to push Him away. We don't like the pain or the discomfort, and instead of seeing all that God is doing in us and for us in the midst of life's difficulty, we fixate on the difficulty and distance from God for allowing it. Jesus had more to say about the world and peace: "Peace I leave with you; my peace I give you. I do not give to you as the world gives. Do not let your hearts be troubled and do not be afraid" (John 14:27 NIV). He says that the world will dish out problems, but that He has overcome the world. When we spend time in His presence, we build the trust to believe that is true. We can experience the peace He wants to give us, a peace that will keep our hearts from being troubled and afraid.

## Praying to My Enlightened Self

Trending media doesn't just encourage us to pray to the universe to grant us our every whim (providing that we speak positively enough). There has been and continues to be popular enticement to pray to our enlightened selves. To make ourselves the center of the universe, the holder of all wisdom and the answer to all of life's problems, seems narcissistic at best and a scary proposition for all of us involved at the worst. That philosophy presumes an arrogance that flies in the face of dependence on God for help and guidance. I (Linda) don't know about you, but in my most eloquent moments, with my most competent comprehensions, trying my dead-level best, I am still a hot mess compared to the hope and healing that God provides and continues to make available to all who ask.

Praying to my past or future self not only defies logic, but it presumes a level of self-importance often embraced by folks who don't want to be accountable to anyone for their life choices. Our accountability to the Lord is for our benefit, and the precepts He has laid out for us in the Bible offer us a template to live by that provides us with a life that flourishes.

In today's culture, we like the idea of being spiritual people but without the burden of obedience that will bring abundant life. Google reports that the word *spirituality* is searched over 350,000 times a month. *Spiritual* is searched 2,700,000 in the same amount of time. According to a six-year study completed by the Barna Research Group, while more than two-thirds of Americans say that are either "religious" or "spiritual," they admit to not being committed to faith matters. The study states, "At times Americans put a positive face on their reason for being; other times they admit to not living up to their ideals. For instance, while 71% of adults believe they are 'fulfilling their calling in life,' 51% also say they are 'searching for meaning and purpose.'"[3]

God gives us life-changing meaning and purpose when we surrender to His will for us and live the life He lays out for us in His Word. We won't find it by making our own rules. Just look at today's world: The further we drift from the laws of the Lord, the more of a mess we become.

If we are connected to the world's wisdom, only a click away, we have to balance that with connection to our wise and worship-wor-

---

3 "American Spirituality Gives Way to Simplicity and the Desire to Make a Difference" Barna Research, Faith and Christianity, January 28, 2009: https://www.barna.com/.../american-spirituality-gives-way-to-simplicity-and-the-desire-t...

thy God. It means turning off our digital connections and tuning in to our divine one.

With the help of the apostle Paul, I developed a tool to help us move away from the clutter of the world and the anxiety that accompanies that clutter and into the presence of our competent Christ. I call it **The Formula from Philippians 4**. It has helped Bev and me personally, and we have used it with countless people whom we have counseled to help them as well. But it needs to be done with focus and intentionality, and we know how hard that can be in this tech-pecked culture. Without intentionality, we can busily offer up a prayer, say amen, and head out to tackle the day on our own—then spend the rest of the day getting knocked down by the challenges life can bring. Let's take a look at the tools found in this Scripture to keep us communicating with God all day long.

## The Formula from Philippians 4

Here are the words of Paul to the Philippians and to us: "Rejoice in the Lord always. I will say it again: Rejoice! Let your gentleness be evident to all. The Lord is near. Do not be anxious about anything, but in every situation, by prayer and petition, with thanksgiving, present your requests to God. And the peace of God, which transcends all understanding, will guard your hearts and your minds in Christ Jesus. Finally, brothers and sisters, whatever is true, whatever is noble, whatever is right, whatever is pure, whatever is lovely, whatever is admirable—if anything is excellent or praiseworthy—think on these things" (Philippians 4:4–8 NIV). Do you want to decompress stress and eliminate anxiety? Do you want the heart-guarding peace this Scripture talks about? Then keep reading.

Shut off your tech devices—all of them—and focus on the concepts that you will see illustrated in the verses you just read.
- Celebration
- Supplication
- Appreciation
- Transformation
- Concentration

In this chapter, we will focus on the first three, and here is how you can remember the tool. When you are not clinging to your phone, you can hold up your unencumbered hand and extend your five fingers.

Start with your thumb and say the word *Celebration*. Associate each word with another finger. Lifting your index finger, you will think about the word *Supplication.* Next is the middle finger, and the word *Appreciation* (certainly a better expression than is so often used in today's anxiety-ridden world, don't you think?). Raising the ring finger, say the word *Transformation.* Finish your recitation with the pinkie and then think about the word *Concentration*. When the day rolls in with irritation, frustration, and stress, hold up your hand and review this template to keep you connected to Christ.

Let's look deeper at the benefits provided for us in our **Formula from Philippians 4.**

## Celebration (Your Thumb)

In Paul's words to the Philippians we read, "Rejoice in the Lord always; again I will say, rejoice!" (Philippians 4:4 NIV). I can almost hear Paul, the passionate preacher, saying, "Rejoice in the Lord. That bears repeating. I'll say it again—rejoice!" No matter how challenging life is, we always have something to rejoice about, and that's important to remember on taxing days.

It's easy to be consumed with the challenge that is on the road ahead of us, but if we take an inventory of how far we've come and all that God has done, it fuels our faith to keep going. Paul wasn't the only author in the Bible who understood the value of celebrating God's goodness. David made it a pattern in his life to praise, as we see in Psalm 146:1–2: "Praise the LORD. Praise the LORD, O my soul! I will praise the LORD all my life; I will sing praise to my God as long as I live." There are times when praise effervesces from us as we view a beautiful sunrise, a friend's kind words, or a baby's laugh. Then there are times when praise is the last thing in the world we want to do. But David continues to encourage us in Psalm 103:1–5: "Praise the Lord, O my soul; all my inmost being, praise his holy name. Praise

118

the Lord, O my soul, and forget not all his benefits—who forgives all your sins and heals all your diseases, who redeems your life from the pit and crowns you with love and compassion, who satisfies your desires with good things so that your youth is renewed like the eagle's" (NIV). Now, that's something to celebrate!

Psalm 103 tells us to "forget not all of his benefits." I (Beverly) am not proud of it, but I can get so busy or so fixated on my plans and worries/concerns, I don't take the time to remember His benefits in my past, and I end up circling the drain, anxious and stressed. Counting my blessings, as the old song goes, helps me to gain a more positive perspective.

In the last chapter, we talked about writing a "Blessed List" and how important it is to help us focus on the positive. Write what's right, then read it regularly, especially if you are going through challenging times. Remembering all that you have been blessed with shifts your perspective from circling the drain to singing God's praises. What's the alternative—tearful, anxious grumbling? Wringing your hands in faithless fear only makes you miserable. Instead, give God praise in spite of your feelings, and He gives you peace in spite of your circumstances.

Paul goes on to say in Philippians 4:5, "Let your gentleness be known to all. The Lord is near" (NIV). When I am mowing through my moments, obsessing about my worries or fretting over the future, I am anything but gentle. I'm harried, irritable, and frustrated, and everyone around me can attest to that! When I celebrate my wins, and I remember that the "Lord is near," I can relax, rest in His presence, and demonstrate gentleness to a world of people looking for hope. (Then my kids won't have to ask, "Where's my mom, and who's the psycho head case that looks like her?") We will demonstrate the gentleness we feel in our trusting hearts because we know God's got it covered.

I want to encourage you that the next time you go to the Lord in prayer burdened for your health or someone else's, your teenager's latest issue, what's not in your wallet, or whatever is weighing you down, go to God with an attitude of celebration before you even present your request. Spend some serious time thanking Him for all the good He has done, then watch how the burden you have on your heart feels lighter even before you ask for His help. While that is good news, we can still ask.

## Supplication (Index Finger)

Philippians 4:6 encourages us, "Be anxious for nothing, but in everything, by prayer and supplication with thanksgiving, let your requests be made known to God" (NASB). In the *Encarta* dictionary, the definition for *supplication* is a "humble request to somebody who has the power to grant the request." God, the Creator of the universe, the One who placed the stars in the heavens and who has numbered every hair on your head (see Matthew 10:30) can handle whatever request we present to Him. Supplication doesn't have to be anxious begging. It's simply focused asking. That's what this new believer experienced.

## Colorful Casey Wayne

Casey Wayne was a self-described mess. He had spent twenty-six years as an angry alcoholic, leaving much human carnage in his path of broken relationships. When he hit his bottom, he was ready to do whatever it took to make the pain go away. He turned his life over to the Lord, started going to recovery meetings, and looked up everyone he could to make amends. He was living the life he had always dreamed of.

Then, on the three-month anniversary of his conversion, he woke up to what he thought later could have been the worst week of his life. His nineteen-year-old son got picked up for his second DUI.

"I blame myself for so much of my son's trouble," Casey Wayne moaned. "I wasn't parenting him. I was at the bottom of a bottle." He tried not to spiral downward in his guilt. Two days later, Casey found out his dad had prostate cancer; it was the same day the company told him they were laying off eight drivers.

"My Bible study group was going through Philippians. When we got to this part about supplication, I knew I needed to give it a try. I didn't have anything to lose except my heavy heart. We all prayed, I gave the Lord my burdens, and I couldn't believe how much peace I had knowing God could handle it all. I didn't have to make myself crazy worrying about all that stuff. In the past, a week like that would have made me drink. Now instead of filling up on booze, I'm filled with the Holy Ghost!" he shared, barely able to contain his enthusiasm.

When we offer up our burdens to the Lord in supplication, it's important that we leave them there. In the last chapter, we took a look at the **Let-Go-and-Let-God Meditation**, which focused on giving God our worries and concerns. Along with Peter's instructions to "cast our cares on the Lord," the psalmist David gave the same advice. Psalm 55:22 instructs us to "cast your cares on the Lord, and he will sustain you; he will never let the righteous to be shaken" (NIV). The word *sustain* in the Hebrew means to provide, to feed, guide, to comprehend.[4] What a comfort to know God gets you. He understands what's going on around you. He understands your concern and your fear, and you don't have to worry about tomorrow. He's already there.

It also means to nurture and to hold. That's a promise to hold on to, pun definitely intended. He comprehends all our concerns, and He apprehends all our fears as He nurtures and holds us. But it gets even better, because the word for *sustain* in Hebrew is spelled *kuwl*. In English, it's pronounced *cool*! We think it is pretty cool, don't you?

You've been where Casey was, haven't you? When you allowed God to have your burden and you actually felt Him take it from you, did you feel His peace? If you haven't done this yet, give it a try. Casey petitioned God to answer his prayer and give him peace, and the Lord did. But God also answers our petitions for others, even when they don't know we are praying.

---

4 Strongs, op.cit., see *sustain*

## Michel's Story

Michel was a tortured adolescent. He was raised in an upper-middle-class family, and he didn't want for anything growing up. But without spiritual moorings to anchor to, like so many, he easily drifted down the river of drugs, alcohol, and poor choices. He tried pot for the first time in the sixth grade. By his sophomore year of high school, he was dropping acid and using anything he could get his hands on.

"When someone asked me what my drug of choice was, I said 'yes,'" he shared in his testimony to a church recovery group. "Even my partying friends were telling me that I partied too much."

Along the way, people invited him to youth group and church. The love and light he felt there was compelling, and there were even brief moments of truly encountering God. But addiction still had its tenacious grip on him. He even dated a youth group girl for a while, but she broke up with him because he wouldn't stop getting drunk.

After high school, he got a job that allowed him to get high every day. After a few encounters with the law, he decided to leave the little town where he lived to party in the big city. So, he headed down to San Diego to stay with his sister and made a plan to meet up with friends and travel to Mexico for an easy score of prescription drugs.

On the third morning he was at his sister's, he opened his eyes and a moment of clarity stabbed him awake. Looking around him, he could palpably feel the hollow emptiness in his chest.

"I have been trying to fill this hole with everything from the deepest drunk to the highest high, but the hole just keeps getting bigger."

And then with the most earth-shattering, soul-saving revelation, he stated, "I need God." He made a plan to head back home to church, to the youth pastor and the friends who were there seeking God. When his druggie buddies showed up to head for Tijuana, he gave them all of his money and his pot and said, "I'm out. I'm done with this." Needless to say, they weren't happy with him but it didn't matter.

He went on: "I found myself breaking all of my CDs. Clearly the music I was listening to was feeding the hopeless darkness in my soul, so I was done with it too.

"I wasn't sure if I was finally figuring life out or having a psychotic episode, but something big was happening in me. I needed a cigarette to cope, so I walked outside to chain-smoke, and just as I did, the marine layer of clouds, that San Diego is so famous for, broke and the sun came beaming through the clouds. As I was soaking in the light, a woman in a bridal gown came walking by. The Southern California coast is a beautiful place for weddings, and she was on her way to hers.

"I looked at her and said out of politeness, 'Nice day.' She looked back beaming and said with conviction, 'It's the best day ever.' And for the first time in as long as I could remember, I felt like it was.

"I went to the bus station and somehow ended up on the wrong bus. At least that's what I thought. For God's purposes in me, it wasn't the wrong bus. I ended up traveling through the roughest parts of Los Angeles, with homeless drug addicts on every corner. I kept hearing in my head, *This is where you were heading,* and I knew that was the sobering truth.

"I arrived back home at 2 a.m., and my faithful mom was there to pick me up. In the midst of all of my issues, she had found her way to God. So, her first words were, 'Do you want to come with me to church tomorrow?'

"My youth pastor, Peter, met me as I came up the aisle of church, and it felt like a scene from Luke 15, where the dad comes out to meet the prodigal when he finally gets a clue and comes home. Pete told me that he and some of the kids in the youth group came to my work to look for me because they hadn't seen me in a while. When my boss said I had left town, they stopped right in front of the restaurant where I got high every day and prayed that I would come to God and back to church.

"On my first day back to the youth group, Pete had me share with everyone in the room the story of what had just happened to me. They prayed for me and supported me, and I finally felt that sense of belonging my soul was craving.

"Several weeks passed and the girl I dated, the one who had dumped me for staying drunk, came up to me. Someone who had heard me tell my story shared it with her. She had just come back from a Youth With A Mission school where she had spent three solid months investing in her relationship with God.

"One night as the students were in a prayer meeting, one of her fellow students approached her and said, 'I have a word for you, a message that I believe is straight from God for you. You have a friend; he has red hair. You know who he is. He needs prayer right now, and it's a matter of life and death.' So my friend prayed for me and asked the students who didn't even know me, and they prayed that I could get out of Satan's clutches and finally fully give myself to God. Then my friend opened up her journal to show me that all this had happened on the very day I was in San Diego finally figuring life out!"

Today Michel is as fine and refined as a young man can get. He has served as a youth pastor for the last fifteen years at a growing church, and because of his faithfulness and skill, he has moved up the ranks to associate pastor, a role in which he preaches the Word, looks out for God's people, and seeks to help anyone who is looking for God like he was.

I often wonder where Michel would be now if those folks hadn't taken seriously this incredible gift of calling out to the Lord on his behalf. Michel's soul would not have been the only one lost. The hundreds of people that he has impacted through his ministry over the years would have been affected as well. Now that truth stabs me awake and gets me on my knees to stay faithful in prayer.

## Appreciation (Middle Finger)

As we read Philippians 4:6, "Do not be anxious about anything, but in every situation, by prayer and petition, with thanksgiving, present your requests to God" (NIV), we can't look past the two words in the middle of the verse. They give us a key instruction for staying connected with Christ. Those words are *"with thanksgiving."* While we are laying out our requests to the Lord, we must stay in gratitude. Continuing to thank God shifts our focus to what we have, rather than keeping it on what we don't.

In this indulgent culture, we can easily move from appreciation to expectation. As parents, we find ourselves troubled with how kids lack gratitude, don't we? They really don't know how good they've got it, as they continue to take all they have been given for granted. It seems that every generation has its version of this message. I'm sure our parents said this about our generation, too, at some point. If we aren't careful, we can do the same thing to God. We can complain our way through life and take for granted all of God's amazing provision unless we cultivate an attitude of gratitude.

Take a look at Eve in the Garden of Eden. She had everything she could ask for, but instead of appreciating what she had, she chose to covet what she didn't have. That's our nature. If Eve hadn't messed things up for the human race, you or I likely would have. It takes discipline and intentionality to live in an attitude of gratitude, but the end result is a life of power, no matter what is happening around us.

Appreciation implies trust. First Thessalonians 5:18 instructs us to "give thanks in all circumstances, for this is God's will for you in Christ Jesus" (NIV). Notice it doesn't say to "give thanks for all circumstances." I don't have to say, "Thank You, God, I didn't make a sale today and I have bills to pay." Nor do I have to forfeit my reason and thank God that the doctor told me I have to have surgery. But I must learn to trust what His Word shows me in verses like Isaiah 41:10: "So do not fear, for I am with you; do not be dismayed, for I am your God. I will strengthen you and help you; I will uphold you with My righteous right hand" (NIV). If I can remember all the times He has provided for and comforted me, I can stay positive. His nature demonstrates that He will do that again and again. So, even in the dark times, I can focus on His light, knowing that His mercies are new every morning (see Lamentations 3:22–24).

As we move through our template embracing **Celebration** and **Supplication** with **Appreciation,** we will find ourselves moving in the direction toward **Transformation** and the heart-guarding peace that God promises. Let's see what that looks like.

## Making It Real

1. Do you agree that the more time we spend investing in something, the more influence it has on us? How much is your life influenced by your digital dependence?

2. Is it possible that you could spend less screen time and have more meaningful time each day? Write about what that would look like.

3. Do you find that media has influenced your belief systems? How?

4. Do you seek to make God's Word the bedrock of your belief system, or can you see how digital influence has played a part? What values, ideals, and pursuits need to be amended in order to reflect a biblical worldview?

5. What steps can you take to make the Bible your standard for living? (For example: Read the Word daily. Allow it to dictate your views and decisions, even if that flies in the face of current trends. Pray for the Lord to keep you strong and to influence the rest of the world to embrace Him and His teachings. More?)

Chapter 12

# Brain Change

The digital age has radically increased the amount of information our brains have to process in a single day. As people, we are programmed to respond to all of the information coming at us, and that stimulus overload is too much to handle. It creates what researchers call "Busy Brain Syndrome": "Busy Brain is 'maladaptation' of brain processing because of the overload of sensory bombardment due to technology increasing the amount of 'stuff' the brain has to deal with at any time. It is not digital intrusion—it is the downstream effect of digital intrusion changed brain capacity."[1]

## Busy Brain Syndrome

Busy Brain Syndrome causes a shutdown in the prefrontal cortex, the executive function of the brain, leaving the less-finessed part of our brain—the fight, flight, or freeze function—to kick in to deal with a perceived threat. In this state of stress, the adrenal glands release more cortisol. This is known as the limbic system, and it is designed by God to protect us from danger. The problem is that this lower, or more primitive, part of the brain is immature, subjective, highly emotional, and reactive.

The activation of the limbic system interferes with our ability to assimilate information, lowers our immune function and bone den-

---

1 Debbie Hampton, "Four Steps to Take Control of your Mind and Change Your Brain," *The Best Brain Possible*, June 5, 2016: https://www.thebestbrainpossible.com/four-steps-to-take-control-of-your-mind-and-change-your-brain/

sity, and can lead to several chronic conditions, such as increased weight gain, high cholesterol, and heart disease.

With stimuli coming at us at lightning speed, our stressed-out state has become a default setting, creating a constant dump of cortisol into our systems. According to mental health specialist Dr. Barbara Mariposa, this physiological stress response causes us to react as though "we have an accelerator pedal on our adrenal glands, set at full throttle leaving us running on empty with no reserve. Our tension is further fueled by the fear that if we actually did unplug we would be rendered ineffective and unproductive, or worse actually fall apart."[2]

Without the logic that the prefrontal cortex provides, we end up stuck in a negative mind-set, obsessing on negative thoughts and feelings. The end result is a group of anxious, edgy, foggy-brained, sickly people who operate at less-than-optimal levels on any task they attempt. Globally the quality of life is the highest it's ever been, but so are our rates of anxiety and depression.

If we continue to live tech-pecked, we will remain in a constant state of stress as our bodies keep score. We can even become so programmed to listen for every ping, ding, or buzz that we actually think we are hearing them when they aren't even present (also known as Phantom Text Syndrome). Talk about anxiety!

I (Beverly) actually experienced this as I was writing this book. My main computer got infected with a virus, so I began working with an older model that did not have the features that made editing easy. I missed my newer computer so much that I found myself anxiously listening to my phone as I waited for the repair company to call. I jumped at every buzz, real or imagined, which only heightened my anxiety, not to mention the toll it took on my creative process. I had to recommit to the tools we had researched for this book so that I could move back to a mental place of optimal productivity and contentment.

The tools we continue to present are designed to help all of us, in this age of information, to unplug for long enough periods of time

---

2 Hampton, ibid.

to give our brains and bodies time to recoup. When we decide not to live tech-pecked, with constant interruptions, and we choose to turn off to tune in, we won't live in constant fight-or-flight mode. Our prefrontal cortex will remain in charge of our responses, and our efficiency, along with our overall well-being, will improve.

We can choose what we allow our brains to focus on even when we are being bombarded with negative and intrusive thoughts. Scripture tells us that we are transformed by the renewing of our minds. Our thoughts don't have to dictate our actions. We can rule over our thoughts.

Here is the scriptural proof: "And so, dear brothers and sisters, I plead with you to give your bodies to God. Let them be a living and holy sacrifice—the kind he will accept. When you think of what he has done for you, is this too much to ask? Don't copy the behavior and customs of this world, but let God transform you into a new person by changing the way you think. Then you will know what God wants you to do, and you will know how good and pleasing and perfect his will really is" (Romans 12:1–2 NLT). The Lord can help us change the way we think. It may not be easy, but with determination, repetition, and the power of the Holy Spirit, we can choose not to be controlled by our flawed perspectives. We can be transformed.

That brings us to the rest of our template. Using your hand to remember and embrace the tools of **Celebration, Supplication, and Appreciation** will pave the way for the kind of **Transformation** that this passage in Romans describes.

## Transformation (Ring Finger)

Philippians 4:7 promises us power that can be hard for us to fathom. Here we are in the midst of our demanding days with challenges at every turn, and we can experience unexplainable peace. Talk about transformation!

Let's read those words again: "And the peace of God, which transcends all understanding, will guard your hearts and your minds in Christ Jesus" (NIV). Don't we all long for that kind of peace? With-

129

out it we can go from zero to crazy in thirty seconds flat. However, when we move through the **Formula from Philippians 4**, we can feel supernatural transformation as the Lord brings us to a place of peace and stands as a sentry by our heart's door to keep out the craziness so that we can stay there.

You've seen that look of unexplainable peace in the woman whose husband just lost his job, and she surprises herself with how calmly she reacts. You have witnessed it in the pastor who just buried his brother and his father within three weeks of each other. Still, you see an amazing peace in his eyes. You find it in the church saint awaiting another test for possible cancer, and she's the one encouraging those who love her. Perhaps you've experienced it yourself. You look at all you have on your plate, and you marvel at how you aren't falling apart.

## Shelley's Story

Time spent in the Lord's presence leads to transformation. That's what Shelley discovered. Her world nearly collapsed when her husband walked out on her and their two boys. "I don't know what I'm going to do," she sobbed, sitting on the plaid sofa of my office. "Derek is gone, and he's not coming back. He's moved in with this secretary. She's practically a child. Ethan and Ryan are crushed and want nothing to do with their dad. He keeps inviting them over, and he's clueless as to why they won't come. Can he not see how they feel betrayed that he broke up our family? Are they just supposed to go over and hang out at Dad's with his girlfriend, who doesn't seem much older than they are, and act like nothing's wrong? What's he thinking?"

"He's not thinking. That's the problem," I (Linda) informed.

"I feel so inadequate. I've been traded in for a newer model because I've got too many miles on me, miles that taking care of Derek helped to put there," she moaned.

I nodded to affirm her feelings and keep her opening up. Her honesty was helping her get to the root of her issues. Stuffing her feelings would only make them fester.

"I'm going to have to sell the house, and it's the only home the boys have known. Then I'm going to have to go to work. I haven't had a job in ten years. Derek never wanted me to work so I would have time to run his errands and make home-cooked meals. So, I dutifully complied—for all the good it did me." She drew in a ragged breath and kept talking.

"Linda, why did God let this happen? He could have made Derek wake up," she sighed with a resignation that let me know she had dumped all she could for the moment.

"I believe God tried. If your husband ever comes out of his 'love coma,' and if he's being honest, he will admit that God made efforts to get through to him. Shelley, God is limited by only one thing. He's not limited by evil. He's not restricted by Satan. Jesus doesn't sweat Satan. He's limited only by our will, because He loves us enough to let us choose. I believe He goes to great lengths to engineer a path to help us choose wisely, but ultimately, we are the ones who make the choice. Derek made his choice, and it is not without consequences.

"It is hard to suffer pain from someone who is supposed to love you. Try not to run their dad down in front of them, even though Derek has earned their disapproval and they are deeply hurt by him. It will take time for him to win back their favor. In the meantime, you are going to have to take care of you. You've made a career out of caring for everyone else. Now it's time to put you on that list.

"You can be angry with God right now, because that's real. Have your fit and fall in it, as they say in the South, but be ready to move on when it's over, because it's not God's fault. The best friend you have right now is the Lord. We're going to spend the rest of this hour praying through those angry feelings so you can embrace His power and peace for the days ahead."

I led her through a prayer exercise to help her to dump her baggage of resentment, grief, and self-loathing, and a smile emerged from all of those tears.

"We have more bags to unpack," I informed her, "but this should start you on your path to healing."

"I feel tired but lighter," she confessed.

131

"I'm glad you were able to dump some of your burden. Shelley, I have a word of caution for you. Right now, since you are still dealing with anger toward Derek, questioning God, and needing to prove you are desirable, it would be easy to go out and do something unwise that you will regret forever. That would blow up your life right now. You would not believe the good Christian women who do that because of momentary lapses in judgment at times like these. Hang in there. You might not believe me right now, but you will feel better sooner than you think."

"After our prayer, I'm already feeling better," she informed me.

"And that's your secret weapon," I continued. "If you're tempted to 'do stupid,' get on your knees."

We both laughed, and she promised she would do that.

Shelley stayed the course, continuing to go to church and attend counseling sessions to keep her heart focused on Christ. She even joined a women's Bible study and let the ladies of the church love on her. That came in handy the day after Derek showed up at Ryan's soccer game with his new young girlfriend.

"Ryan was so upset he left the field without speaking a word to his dad. Derek accused me of putting him up to that. He still doesn't get the damage he's doing." Shelley shook her head. "Thank God for the ladies in my Bible study group who let me cry and prayed for me."

One of the women in her Bible study helped her get a part-time job. Another lady kept an eye on Ethan until Ryan got home from high school each day. "It's certainly not easy by any means, but I do feel like God is directing my steps," Shelley admitted one afternoon in counseling.

"Keep claiming God's promises and keep hanging in. You're experiencing God's transforming power even when it's hard. I'm proud of you," I assured her.

Shelley did hang in there, and three years after Derek left, she met Ed, a wonderful Christian man who started attending her small group at church. He fell in love with her and her sons. They were married a year later.

Shelley was stunning at the wedding. At the reception, she came over to my table and gave me a big hug. Beaming from ear to ear, she offered, "God is so good, Linda," realizing I knew exactly what she meant.

Shelley's heart was transformed from a fearful fretter to a faith-filled follower, even under the most anxious of circumstances. Addiction to worry and fear can be crippling for sure, but perhaps your addiction feels more damaging.

## Tech and Addiction

We can't write a book about being tech-pecked without addressing how technology has created an entirely new addictive process. With a single click, a world of sexual images can hold a person captive and it's hard to escape the lure. With digital devices in the palm of our hands, porn addiction has become epidemic. A recent study conducted over the past five years reveals that 68 percent of Christian men view porn on a regular basis, with the biggest users between the ages of 11 and 17 years old. Those are staggering statistics.

Addiction is consuming, and those trapped by it know how difficult it is to shed its tenacious grip. But it can happen. Eighty-four years of Alcoholics Anonymous and twenty-seven years of Celebrate Recovery, not to mention all the other effective recovery programs that are available, prove that with work and help from our Higher Power, we can recover. When we replace, "I can't," with "By the Lord's power, I can," it works. When we attend meetings to continue to hear the truth about who we are and let that truth renew our minds, and when we seek accountability and support in that group, we can find healing. "It works if you work it," is a common mantra among those walking in new light on a daily basis.

Whether it is technology, FOMO, chronic worry, alcohol, anxiety, pornography, or something else, we do not have to be held hostage by our bad habits. God gives us the awesome power to be transformed. However, without concentrating on Him, we can easily forget all we have learned.

## Concentration (Pinkie Finger)

Philippians 4:8–9 instructs us, "Finally, brothers and sisters, whatever is true, whatever is noble, whatever is right, whatever is pure, whatever is lovely, whatever is admirable—if anything is excellent or praiseworthy—think about such things" (NIV).

What we focus on makes a difference. I can obsess about my problems and pound through my day hoeing my negative row. Then my day doesn't end up well for anyone, least of all me. But when I focus with intentionality on the things Paul presents in this verse, it is easier for me to stay in a place of grace.

The best way I know to concentrate on what is true, noble, right, pure, lovely, admirable, excellent, and praiseworthy is to spend time in talking to God in prayer and to open His Word. Prayer helps us keep our minds focused, and Scripture is the truth that sets us free from our crippling hurts, hang-ups, and habits.

## Practicing What I Preach

God consistently presents opportunities for me to practice what I (Linda) preach. God called the **Formula from Philippians 4** to my recollection at a time when I really needed it. It had to be God, because my attitude was so negative, I would have never gotten there without His gentle whisper.

I had just returned from a trip back East, and I was working hard playing catch up with my clients and chores around the house. I was scheduled to speak in Detroit that following weekend, and I was feeling the pressure of a packed schedule.

After viewing the news that night, my husband shared an article with me about the Hanta virus. It had killed several people in Yosemite National Park, less than an hour away from us. We realized from the pictures that the carrier was the same kind of mouse we had seen nesting all over our property—in the sheds and the garage. We even found several of the mice building nests on the radiator of each of our cars!

Realizing how deadly the virus was—there was only a 65 percent chance of survival, even if it was caught early—we went on the warpath. My husband attacked the tiny shed that held our water softener, but the next morning he woke up with a raging headache and flulike symptoms. I was horrified, so off he went to the doctor, while I readied myself to tackle the task at hand. Thank God he only had the flu, but his illness only reinforced my determination.

I suited up with a mask, gloves up to my elbows, and armed with my spray bottle of bleach, I pulled everything out of the garage. I sprayed, scrubbed, soaked, slopped, sopped, and mopped everything in sight. But the process was like pulling a thread. One project led to another, and every time I pulled something out of the garage, I had that much more mess to tackle.

Cleaning consumed my weekend, only by then there was stuff from the garage all over the front yard. Only half the garage was clean, and I had a busy week of counseling and my trip to Detroit the next weekend, where I was to speak four times at a retreat. The mess all over my front yard was an itch I had to scratch until the job was finished. Despite my best efforts to stay positive, the project kept me awake, and I fought hard to stay positive and not descend into cranky until things were put back in order.

I headed into my week cleaning every minute I wasn't working, and by Wednesday I was weary. I had a hard day of counseling, and as I was packing up my things to head home to my lawn, which looked the aftermath of a pauper's yard sale, strewn with everything from lawn chairs to Christmas lights, I spotted a notice that I was to report for jury duty the following day. I had all but forgotten it because in all the years I had received notices, I had always been called off. Now, I want to do my civic duty for the community, but this was not the day for it. In the past, I'd called the number listed on the jury duty notice to find out the case had been settled and my services would not be required. I had assumed that would be the case this time. I had assumed wrong. I was scheduled to report at 8:45 the next morning.

I immediately got on the phone to reschedule all of Thursday's appointments, which was no easy task. Now weary, worn, and irritated, I fumed all the way home. "I can't believe this," I thought to myself. "The last thing in the world I need is one more thing on my plate." After fuming for the rest of the evening about how I didn't need this new headache, I finally decided to go to bed early. I breathed a halfhearted prayer asking God to help my attitude and to give me the self-control to be nice to the folks at the courthouse the next day.

God even hears halfhearted prayers. The next morning, He reminded me of the **Formula from Philippians 4**. I have to give God credit, because I was in a mood. If it had been left up to me, I would have complained all the way there and taken out my frustration on anyone who crossed my path.

As I got in the car, I put my phone on silent so that I could spend some uninterrupted time with the Lord. The last thing I needed was to be tech-pecked to pieces after the past few days of anxious stress. That allowed my heart to be quiet enough to hear the still, small voice of the Lord. He brought to my awareness all the things that were good in my life. My husband didn't have the Hanta virus, and I was healthy enough to tackle the project of making sure that neither of us would get it. That was clearly a cause for **Celebration**. No longer grousing, I noticed what a beautiful day it was. I was driving to the courthouse by a beautiful lake near our house, not into a busy city. I praised the Lord for the beauty around me, and as I celebrated, I felt my mood beginning to shift.

Then I laid my needs out before the Lord with **Supplication**. Asking Him for the power to handle the days ahead, I felt His strength in my weakness. That was cause for **Appreciation**, and I thanked God as I drove. Moving more into appreciation, I realized that I wasn't going to the doctor, or to visit a loved one who was laid up in the hospital. I wasn't driving to a difficult surgery appointment; it was only to jury duty.

My appreciation was allowing me to feel God's **Transformation** as I was getting all up in that peace thing that Philippians talks about. To seal the deal, I moved to **Concentration** as I focused the truth of His Word to help me stay in that place of empowered peace. I reviewed one of my favorite passages from Paul as he quoted God's message to him, that the Lord's strength is made perfect in our weakness. Here is that passage in its entirety: "But he said to me, 'My grace is sufficient for you, for my power is made perfect in weakness.' Therefore I will boast all the more gladly about my weaknesses, so that Christ's power may rest on me. That is why, for Christ's sake, I delight in weaknesses, in insults, in hardships, in persecutions, in difficulties. For when I am weak, then I am strong" (2 Corinthians 12:9–10 NIV). I didn't stop there. I recited 2 Timothy 1:7: "For God did not give us a spirit of timidity, but of power, and love and discipline" (NASB). I was feeling the peace, and it was **transforming** me.

By the time I got to my destination, my bad attitude had lifted. I felt empowered for a great day, and as they ushered us into the courthouse searching everything but the fillings in our teeth, I didn't grumble at anyone and wreck my Christian witness! As I waited to be called, I found a quiet corner and opened my laptop. I could actually focus on what I was studying for the talks I was giving the following weekend because I wasn't wallowing in self-pity because of my perceived bad luck. All of the research I had been reading for this project led me to turn off the alerts on my email as well as my phone. Without digital distractions, I was able to embrace "*unifocus*," a word that has been made necessary in today's culture because of the damage that multitasking is doing to our brains. I really got "in the zone" and was able to fully concentrate and get so much accomplished in a short period of time.

I was slow to realize that God had this day planned out for me. I finished up my writing and contemplated grabbing my phone to check out Facebook when I caught myself. Instead, I looked around for a real-live person to be "social" with. About that time, a couple of sisters I knew from church rounded the corner heading for the bathroom. I hadn't seen them in a while, and we had a delightful visit. Before they left, the older sister expressed to me her desire to get back to regular church attendance.

As the sisters walked away, a lady come to herd all of us into the courtroom, where she promptly announced that the judge was letting us all go! It was 11 a.m. I had cancelled my appointments, so I had the rest of the day to rest and finish putting my garage back in order. Instead of pouting about the inconvenience like I would have done without God's divine reminder, I praised the Lord for His goodness all the way home, realizing the great things He had planned for my day all along.

When I arrived back home, I sat down with a glass of iced tea for few quiet moments on the deck to celebrate my transformation with the Lord, before I completed the task I had started nearly a week before. By the time my husband arrived home from work, the garage was clean, so was I, and we had a chance to spend a quiet evening together before I caught a plane out of town the next morning. I continued my appreciation for the Lord throughout the evening, thankful for the reminder of the **Formula from Philippians 4** that had kept me from fretting away a great day in frustration.

The Lord can transform us if we keep our focus on Him. That's a lot more doable when we temper our tech use. We will explore more ways to do that in the next chapter.

## Making It Real

1. Do you suffer from Busy Brain Syndrome? What will you do about it? (For example: Set boundaries with tech use, eliminate alerts, set aside times to unplug, and more...)

2. Be honest with yourself. Are you addicted to pornography? Seek out a counselor and/or find a recovery group near you, such as Celebrate Recovery, the Conquer Series, or others.

3. Review the verses from the **Formula from Philippians** 4:7. Philippians 4:4–7 says, "Rejoice in the Lord always. I will say it again: Rejoice! Let your gentleness be evident to all. The Lord is near. Do not be anxious about anything, but in every situation, by prayer and petition, with thanksgiving, present your requests to God. And the peace of God, which

transcends all understanding, will guard your hearts and your minds in Christ Jesus" (NIV). Write out your reflections on this section of Scripture.

4. Have you ever experienced a time in your life when you had to hang on to your belief that God was taking care of things over a long period of time, like Shelley did? Did you get to a place of heart-guarding peace? Describe that situation.

5. Do you, like most of us, need divine intervention to help you concentrate on the words and ways of the Lord? Write a note and post it in an obvious place (on your desk, mirror, refrigerator...) to remind you to ask God to help you concentrate on Him. Put it where you will read it often.

6. Has the Lord ever intervened for you even when your attitude didn't deserve His favor? Write about it.

# Chapter 13

# Living Tech-Pecked or Tuned In

In a recent story for ABC News, dated July 27, 2018, Dr. Nancy Cheever, a researcher from California State University, Dominguez Hills, stated, "If you're feeling down and mentally tired, your phone—which is probably always on and in your pocket—might be the problem." Her new study has linked anxiety, severe depression, suicide attempts, and suicide with the growing use of smartphones and other devices.

Cheever states, "The more people use their phone, the more anxious they are about using their phone." Her research suggests that phone-induced anxiety operates on a positive feedback loop, saying that phones keep us in a persistent state of anxiety, and the only relief from this anxiety is to look at our phones. "If you're constantly connected, you're going to feel anxiety," Cheever said. "And the more people feel anxiety, that can lead to other things like mental health and physical ailments."[1]

This can be particularly damaging for teens. Her research comes at a time when young people may be on their phones for more than six and a half hours a day, according to the nonprofit Common Sense Media.

1 Nancy Cheever, "Excessive Cellphone Use May Cause Anxiety, Experts Warn," *ABC News,* July 28, 2017: https://abcnews.go.com/Lifestyle/excessive-cellphone-anxiety-experts-warn/story?id...

"These days, teens can never just step away from their social lives," said Brian Nolan, guidance director at a secondary school in Illinois. "When your parents were at school, they could hang out with their friends during the day, and they would relax with their family at night. There was some kind of balance. But the smart-phone doesn't give you that break. The constant fear of missing out, or the urge to feel included, keeps teens connected. When students only interact via technology, they're much more likely to withdraw from healthier interactions, and are more likely to be hypersensitive to what's being posted. If they aren't included, they can feel lonely. If they are included, they can feel pressure to keep up."

Nolan added, "Parents are not much help because they them-selves are showing children that the phone is more important, when they stop conversations to deal with a text or a WhatsApp message."[2]

Social worker Allison Bean states, "Teens are physically isolating themselves more and more from their real support systems during a time of their lives that can be very stressful. They are depriving themselves of the opportunity to exercise their social skills; skills that are critical for life. It stops students from leaving their rooms to interact with [people of the same age] in a developmentally appro-priate way."[3]

Rian Rowles, chairman of psychiatric services at Advocate Christ Medical Centre in Illinois, stated, "Bullying used to be something that mainly happened at school, but social media can make it a 24/7 thing."

Rowles continued his observations, "When you're writing and posting things, there's a phenomenon in which you don't have the same filter you might when talking on the phone or in person. I think that lends itself to more abrasive statements," he said. "So not only is it constantly there for these kids, it's more intense."[4]

2 Donna Vickroy, "Technology Triggers Teen Depression," *The Star Online,* January 8, 2018: https://www.thestar.com.my/tech/tech-news/2018/01/08/technology-triggers-teen-depression/
3 Ibid.
4 Ibid.

## Teen Reaction

In an article by the Pew Research Center dated May 31, 2018, teens were given the opportunity to explain their views about the value of social media in their own words. Forty percent of teens said that social media has had a positive impact on their lives, because it helps them keep in touch and interact with others. They make statements like these:

"I think social media has a positive effect because it lets you talk to family members far away." (Girl, age 14)

"I feel that social media can make people my age feel less lonely or alone. It creates a space where you can interact with people." (Girl, age 15)

Others in this group cite the greater access to news and information that social media facilitates (16 percent), or being able to connect with people who share similar interests (15 percent):

"My mom had to get a ride to the library to get what I have in my hand all the time. She reminds me of that a lot." (Girl, age 14)

"It has given many kids my age an outlet to express their opinions and emotions, and connect with people who feel the same way." (Girl, age 15)

Meanwhile, 17 percent of these respondents feel these platforms harm relationships and result in less-meaningful human interactions. Similar respondents think social media distorts reality and gives teens an unrealistic view of other people's lives (15 percent), or that teens spend too much time on social media (14 percent).

"It has a negative impact on social (in-person) interactions." (Boy, age 17)

"It makes it harder for people to socialize in real life, because they become accustomed to not interacting with people in person." (Girl, age 15)

"It provides a fake image of someone's life. It sometimes makes me feel that their life is perfect when it is not." (Girl, age 15)

"[Teens] would rather go scrolling on their phones instead of doing their homework, and it's so easy to do so. It's just a huge distraction." (Boy, age 17)

Another 12 percent criticize social media for influencing teens to give in to peer pressure, while smaller shares express concerns that these sites could lead to psychological issues or drama.[5]

In light of what both the experts and teens have to say about the consumption of digital media, let's explore the possibility of setting boundaries in our tech-obsessed lives.

We can all agree that our digital devices provide so many benefits. They give us up-to-the-minute weather forecasts, play our favorite music, and keep us from getting lost when we visit new vistas. They offer entertainment when we are bored and allow us to talk to people halfway around the world with a simple click. Our phones can be programmed to help us monitor everything from fertility cycles to heart rates. We never miss a moment for a picture because we never have to look for a camera. But if we aren't focused, we might miss all of life's moments as we remain forever married to the screen in front of us, dictated by every ping, ding, or buzz.

Our phones, tablets, and computers have become invaluable to us in our technological age, but they are just tools. We use them, not the other way around. If you are riveted to the worldwide web, setting boundaries may be hard. But we have built a case with current research that provides ample motivation to do just that. Here are some of the steps toward digital detox that we have already mentioned in his book.

## Setting Boundaries with Your Online World

Turn off all unnecessary notifications on your phone. You need to be notified if you get a text, not if one of your friends gets another like.

Get a watch, not a smart watch, and an alarm clock to keep you from using your phone for either telling the time or awakening you in the morning.

Set a time limit each day for Facebook and surfing the net.

Step away from your screens and go outside to soak up nature.

---

5 Monica Anderson and Jingjing Jiang, "Teens, Social Media & Technology," *Pew Research Center,* May 31, 2018: www.pewinternet.org/2018/05/31/teens-social-media-technology-2018/

When you are with a live person, keep your face out of your phone and look instead at his or her face.

Set a time to answer emails each day so that you can focus creatively for periods of time without digital diversions.

Refrain from looking at any screen at least two hours before bedtime.

Examine whether your motivation to be online is to reduce anxiety generated by FOMO, or simply for amusement.

If your motivation to "click on" is anxiety driven, you may need more a prescribed program along with the tools we have already listed. Let's look at a daily strategy for living tuned in and not tech-wrecked.

First, as we have mentioned, move your digital devices out of your bedroom. Charge them in a separate place in your home. When you awaken to an alarm clock, you won't be tempted to chase a news thread down a rabbit hole on CNN or see what post is trending. Instead of opening your computer, open the blinds and enjoy the beauty of the morning. It's important to relocate your charging stations so your digital devices won't be the last things you look at before bed either. Remember the information we presented about blue light's dark side. Looking at a bright screen, however small, just before going to sleep makes the body release approximately 22 percent less melatonin, which is the hormone that triggers sleep, and it will help to guarantee a night of interrupted sleep.

## Be Still Before You Tech-Connect

Before you connect with the virtual world, spend some time with God in the real one. Find a quiet spot for prayer and meditation. Make that your contemplation corner every morning. Utilize the tools we talked about in chapter 10. You will never get to the place of introspection your soul needs if you turn on your devices and enter the never-ending information stream.

If you have been using a Bible app on your phone, buy a hardbound Bible instead. Once you turn on your screen, even if it's to read Scripture, the temptation to scroll may prove too challenging. After you have quieted your heart before the living God for an ample amount of time, you are more ready to tackle the day. Start with at least fifteen minutes; you will find that the behavior brings its own reward and you will hunger for more time in His presence.

If you have trained yourself to check your phone every five minutes, set the timer for every fifteen minutes, as Dr. Rosen suggested in chapter 8. Place your phone facedown and only allow yourself to check it when the alarm goes off. As FOMO becomes less of a tyrant, try setting the alarm for longer stretches of time.[6]

## Tech-Fasts

Set tech-free times each day, especially when you are with your family. Place your phone by the front door when you walk in and purpose in your heart to be fully engaged with the people in your home for the next two hours. The world will survive even if they can't reach you for a couple of hours. If your kids have incorporated your habit of online living, it may not matter that you have disconnected from your i-Life for your real life. You may not have anyone to connect with. That requires more strategy.

When my (Linda's) children were growing up, my husband and I made a considerable effort to make sure our home life was fun. We wanted our kids to want to be with us, because we knew that as adolescence approached, they would need to break away from parental influence. We wanted to assure them that they had a cool place to come home to as they were launching. Our goal was to keep the communication lines open so that they felt safe to talk to us about anything when they needed to. As a result, our dinner table became what we loved to call the "sit down, stand up" time each day. Our kids would regale us with stories of their day with a comedic spin that kept us laughing all evening. Our plan worked. Our kids liked being around us enough to let us influence their adolescence—for the most part.

---

6 Rosen, op.cit. 17.

## Expect Opposition

If you are digitally disconnecting to reconnect with your kids, encourage the entire family to do the same. Expect some serious pushback but be persistent. It takes twenty-one days to change a habit, so don't give up. And most of all, have something fun to engage them—a game or an activity you can do inside or out as weather permits. I know one dad who asks his kids every night to say the best and the worst part of each day. That gets them talking and he learns what's going on in their lives.

Mealtimes are a great time to check in with your kids. Create a no-phone zone at the dinner table. If your family members are in the habit of looking at a screen instead of at each other at a meal, have them put their phones in a basket by the kitchen door. If someone violates that rule, they can do the dishes! This goes without saying that as parents, we have to be examples to our kids. We can't try to correct them if they can't get our attention away from Facebook or calls from work.

## The Need to Connect

Perhaps it has become easier for us to invest in our digital avatars that are permanently pressed, wrinkle-resistant, and cellulite-free than it is to learn how to feel comfortable in our own skin. We've grown used to feeling the pull of perceived popularity by the number of likes our posts receive rather than investing in the love we get from eye-to-eye, knee-to-knee conversations.

In an article entitled "FaceTime: The Analogue Version," author Orianna Fielding writes, "As human beings we have a primal need to touch and feel and connect in a real way. We have to remember that within us is a fundamental human desire to feel emotion face-to-face and not just through a digital filter. It is important to engage our five senses again and start to touch things other than a digital device. We thrive on facial feedback, as emotionally this gives us a sense of well-being through oxytocin being released by the brain.

147

We need to stop finding ways, through digital distraction to avoid physical contact."[7]

As counselors who spend a great deal of time helping couples learn better ways to communicate, we are more than surprised by the number of couples who rely on texting as their primary form of communication. We have known and taught for years that communication is only 7 percent the words themselves. Thirty-eight percent is pace, pitch, and tone, and the rest is body language. Hence, texting causes couples to miss out on most of the connection process.

## The Effects of Texts

Lori Schade and Jonathan Sanberg, researchers at Brigham Young University in Utah, conducted a study of the social effects of text messaging. Their research showed that an overuse of texting can actually disconnect couples as it removes the subtlety from a relationship. The study surveyed 276 young adults across the United States, 38 percent of whom were in a serious long-term relationship, 46 percent of whom were engaged, and 16 percent of whom were married. The main points the study highlighted were that relying on texting as a primary form of communication in a relationship only allows the expression of a limited, narrow, and one-dimensional view. Although most of the couples surveyed texted each other multiple times day, the study showed that the compressed vocabulary of texts does not allow for the expression of personality or emotion in a way that real conversation does.[8]

Perhaps one of the most challenging downsides of living life online is the current "selfie obsession" and the detriment it poses for teenage girls. The need for peer approval is never higher than it is in the teen years, when sadly, the level of judgment is impaired as the prefrontal cortex is still fully forming. With communication at their fingertips and the deep need to feel popular, young girls—and boys—can post pictures and make comments that can be used

---

7 Orianna Fielding op.cit., 112.
8 Joe Hadfield, "Too much texting can disconnect couples, research finds," *BYU News*, October 30, 2013: https://news.byu.edu/news/too-much-texting-can-disconnect-couples-research-finds

against them later. It's hard to "unsend." The fact that cyberbullying has actually caused suicides in young people is heartbreaking. If they had only stuck around for a few more years, they would have realized how little they really cared about the opinions that controlled them at the time.

That is when an authentic relationship with a caring God pays off. We were able to survive the real-time bullying, belittling, and beatings of our own mother because of the deep faith we forged in our teen years. Our church made all the difference too. It wasn't a Christian community that manipulated with guilt or thrived on shame. We were blessed enough to find a genuine group of Bible-believing folks who loved us like Jesus did. Without a sustainable connection with Christ, we could have easily become more sad statistics.

That brings us to our next chapter, in which we will explore ways to establish a sustainable faith that can be forged with time spent seeking God in quiet, undistracted moments.

## Making It Real

1. School counselor Brian Nolan writes, "If they (teens) aren't included, they can feel lonely. If they are included, they can feel pressure to keep up." Whether you are a teen or not, have you ever fallen prey to this same kind of anxiety? Describe the pressure you feel. Why do you feel this pressure? Or if not, why not?

2. If you are a parent, what can you do to influence your child's use of screen time? We know that values are caught more than they are taught, so what will you do to set an example?

3. List all the positive, valuable uses for your tech connections. Include them all.

4. Now list all the negative influences and habits that your digital connections create. Be thorough. Determine which aspects of your digitally dominated world need revamping.

5. Choose at least four of the suggestions for digital boundaries in this chapter that you can embrace—starting right this minute. Work at them until they become your new normal.

6. If you have been victimized by cyberbullying, then reread the sections of this book that will help you press into a rewarding relationship with a caring and competent God—and know that the next chapter was written with you mind. If you can feel assured that Creator of the universe has your back, you will have nothing and no one to fear!

# Chapter 14

# Finding God in an Anxious World

A long with sounding the warning signal for all of us to keep from selling our souls to silicon, it has been our goal with this book to prove to you, the reader, that there is a God who loves you with an unfailing love, and that He desires to have a close personal relationship with the person sitting in your seat. But if the devices in our digitally dominated world consume the majority of our time and mental energy, when will we find the space in our lives to tune in to God? "We seemed to have reached a point where we willingly trade real communication and human contact for a piece of hardware. A smartphone does not breathe, or have a pulse or think, but we often give it more attention than we give our partners, children, and work colleagues. We give it power by allowing it to monopolize our time, our thoughts and our relationships.... We have been carried along by a digital wave of change and as a consequence we seem to have lost our ability to experience life in real time. We have lost the ability to find the 'spaces in between,' filling them instead with digital noise. Managing our digital lives seems itself to have almost become a full-time job. We wear 'busyness' as a trophy, but in reality our busyness is not productive. None of us is really 'too busy.' We just need to change the way we prioritize our time and choose living life over digitally editing it on a two-inch screen."[1]

---

1 Fielding, op.cit.116.

As we have presented ideas for monitoring tech use to give you breathing room in your life, we would also like to help you fine-tune your focus as you tune in to the Lord. Here are the stumbling blocks to faith that we have observed in our collective sixty-plus years of counseling. We would like to examine each of these and shed new light if we can.

Perhaps you have a hard time sticking with the idea that God truly exists, and every time you log on to the web, you see more information that He doesn't. Or you believe He exists, but you don't feel worthy of His love or believe that He could conceivably forgive you for all you've done. Maybe you've all but given up on seeking God because your perspective of Him is as the divine taskmaster in the sky. Possibly you have been hurt by the Church or by people who call themselves Christians. Or maybe you earnestly prayed for God to do something and He didn't, so you decided He didn't care. We want to spend some time helping those of you who are wondering about God, or those who are curiously seeking to know about Him. Let's go more in detail with each one of these obstacles to finding God in this digital world.

To dispel doubt, we first have to settle the issue of whether God truly does exist. Even the most stellar of saints can have moments of doubt. Our old pulpit-pounding pastor used to say, "The only people who don't doubt are six feet under." In those moments of skepticism, perhaps this creative metaphor can help you wrap your head around this foundational truth. It resonated with us because it's an anecdotal story about twins, but the deeper inference hits home as well.

## The Tiny Twin Tale

*In a mother's womb were two babies. One asked the other: "Do you believe in life after delivery?" The other replied, "Why, of course. There has to be something after delivery. Maybe we are here to prepare ourselves for what we will be later."*
*"Nonsense," said the first. "There is no life after delivery. What kind of life would that be?" The second said, "I don't know, but there*

*will be more light than here. Maybe we will walk with our legs and eat from our mouths. Maybe we will have other senses that we can't understand now."*

*The first replied, "That is absurd. Walking is impossible. And eating with our mouths? Ridiculous! The umbilical cord supplies nutrition and everything we need. But the umbilical cord is so short. Life after delivery is to be logically excluded."*

*The second insisted, "Well, I think there is something and maybe it's different than it is here. Maybe we won't need this physical cord anymore."*

*The first replied, "Nonsense. And moreover, if there is life, then why has no one ever come back from there? Delivery is the end of life, and in the after-delivery, there is nothing but darkness and silence and oblivion. It takes us nowhere."*

*"Well, I don't know," said the second, "but certainly we will meet Mother, and she will take care of us."*

*The first replied "Mother? You actually believe in Mother? That's laughable. If Mother exists, then where is she now?"*

*The second said, "She is all around us. We are surrounded by her. We are of her. It is in her that we live. Without her, this world would not and could not exist."*

*Said the first: "Well, I don't see her, so it is only logical that she doesn't exist."*

*To which the second replied, "Sometimes, when you're in silence and you focus and listen, you can perceive her presence, and you can hear her loving voice, calling down from above."*[2]

The preborn infant's limited perception of life outside the womb parallels our limited knowledge of life after death. With all of the knowledge that is available in the universe, it seems arrogant to assume with our meager minds that there is no God just because we can't see Him. Then as we examine nature and the intricate complexity of the universe, it seems more of a stretch to believe that

---

2 Voices for Life, "Conversation Between Twins In a Mother's Womb," March 10, 2018, https://thebacajourey.com/two-babies-talking-in-the-womb/

things "just happened" rather than to believe that they were intelligently designed.

We believe and have experienced that the Creator of the universe wants to communicate with and care for those He has created. The last line—"Sometimes, when you're in silence and you focus and listen, you can perceive her presence, and you can hear her loving voice, calling down from above"—illustrates an amazing point. When we idle down, calm our hearts, and quiet our minds, we can hear the Lord speaking to us. In a world that continues to worship sonstant digital dependance, those precious times of hearing from God are few and far between, and that allows our stress, hopelessness, and confusion to continue to grow. As we turn off our tech and tune in to God, we will find our center, our balance, and our reason for being. But so many find it hard to tune in to a God they can't see, and here are some reasons why.

## Feeling Unworthy

Perhaps you have decided that there is a God, a higher power, an intelligent designer, but you just don't know if He could personally love you. You believe God exists, but you dismiss that He is in your corner because you don't feel worthy of a relationship with Him.

If that is how you are feeling, God knew you would be reading this book today, and He wants to settle it with you once and for all. You are valuable to Him—so much so that He would rather die than live without you. There has been a lot of talk in the past few decades about self-esteem. We're talking here about "Jesus-teem," the esteem and value that we accept from the Creator of the universe. If the One who set the stars in the sky and the planets in their orbit loves you, that makes you pretty special, don't you think?

*The Message* translates James 1:16–18 like this: "So, my very dear friends, don't get thrown off course. Every desirable and beneficial gift comes out of heaven. The gifts are rivers of light cascading down from the Father of Light. There is nothing deceitful in God, nothing two-faced, nothing fickle. He brought us to life using the true Word, showing us off as the crown of all his creatures." Everything good that comes into our lives comes from God. This scripture tells us that He isn't fickle; He's not subject to change, like we humans are. He isn't going to wake up in a bad mood and take it out on you. Nor is He an impartial, uncaring entity who plays chess with the universe using you as one of His pawns. He is a loving, capable God who walks with you and who offers hope and peace to all who ask.

## Does God Really Love Me?

There is so much confirmation in God's Word that He loves us with an unquenchable love. In Jeremiah 31:3-4 we read, "The LORD appeared to us in the past, saying: 'I have loved you with an everlasting love; I have drawn you with loving-kindness. I will build you up again...'" (NIV). The New Living Translation uses the word *unfailing* for *everlasting*. They both paint a picture of God's unending love. Perhaps you grew up in home like ours where love always seemed to fail. The unfailing love of the Lord is a compelling proposition and a viable reality if we will embrace it. Zephaniah 3:17 tells us, "For the LORD your God is living among you. He is a mighty savior. He will take delight in you with gladness. With his love, he will calm all your fears. He will rejoice over you with joyful songs" (NLT). God is singing over you—the person reading this book. Soak that up for a minute. Zechariah 2:8 tells us, "For whoever touches you, touches the apple of His (the Lord's) eye" (NIV). Does that make you feel safe and secure? It should.

God declares His love and care in Deuteronomy 33:27: "The eternal God is your refuge, and underneath are the everlasting arms" (NIV). He reinforces that notion in Isaiah 41:13: "For I am the LORD your God, who takes hold of your right hand, who says to you, Do not fear, I will help you" (NIV). He seconds that motion in Romans 5:8: "But God demonstrates His own love toward us, in this: While we were still sinners, Christ died for us" (NIV). Even when we were actively blowing it, Jesus loved us enough to die for us. How much more does He desire to give us now that we are buying a clue and seeking to follow Him? Romans 8:1 informs us, "Therefore there is now no condemnation for those who are in Christ Jesus" (NIV).

## An Unhealthy View of God and Religion

Some people have difficulty seeking relationship with the Lord because they have a skewed view of Jesus and religion. They may associate God with duty and diligence and miss those parts in His Word that confirm His acceptance and compassion.

Whether we get the idea from growing up in legalistic churches, being raised by rigid parents, or concocting our own distorted ideas of the Almighty, we can end up with the notion that God is the relentless taskmaster in the sky. Then when we feel unhappy with our performance or upset with our own actions, we project our disappointment with ourselves onto God and decide that He disapproves of us. So, we pull away from Him while blaming Him for the distance between us. The end result is that we either try harder on our own to be good enough, or we give up on God altogether. Think about it—like we could ever do or be good enough to earn the gift of Christ's death on the cross for all the poor choices we have made in our lives. What could any of us ever do to deserve such favor? Nothing, but He offers it to us anyway.

## Feelings of Guilt and Shame

Often people distance from God because they don't feel forgiven for their sins. Let's get "down and dirty," or rather I (Linda) should say, let's get "clean" about confessed sin. First John 1:9 reads, "If we confess our sins, he is faithful and righteous to forgive us our sins and to cleanse us from all unrighteousness" (NIV). It doesn't say *some* unrighteousness; it says *all* unrighteousness. Psalm 103:12 explains, "As far as the east is from the west, so far has he removed our transgressions from us" (NIV). God informs us in Hebrews 8:12, "For I will forgive their wickedness and will remember their sins no more" (NIV). After we confess our sins to the Lord, He is done with them; we don't have to live with guilt or spend our lives running from God for fear that He will find out who we are and press His divine *smite* button to wreck us for all eternity. The Bible tells us in Psalm 103:8–10, "The LORD is compassionate and gracious, slow to anger, abounding in love. He will not always accuse nor will he harbor his anger forever; he does not treat us as our sins deserve, nor repay us according to our iniquities" (NIV). The Lord forgives us for our sins, so we owe it to ourselves to do the same.

The word for "sin" in the New Testament is the word *hamartano*. It means "to miss the mark." In John 8, when the high-and-mighty religious leaders brought a woman caught in adultery to Jesus, they wanted to trick Jesus with just what you are struggling with too. Jesus preached love and grace, and here was a woman clearly messing up, caught in the very act of sin. They really thought they had Him. I love Christ's response to this struggling sinner. After He put her accusers in their place, He didn't unleash his wrath on her. The Bible doesn't record the holy God-Man telling her what a disappointing sinner she was. He didn't condemn her, but He knew she was missing the mark, missing God's best for her life. So, He told her to go and "sin no more." He encouraged her to aim higher. Perhaps all this troubled woman needed was for someone to believe she actually could.

Still, it's a tall order to aim higher, but we don't have to do that on our own power. We can ask the Holy Spirit to do it in us. Remember what Paul tells us in Philippians 2:13: "For God is working in you, giving you the desire and the power to do what pleases Him" (NLT). Not only will God give us the power to make good choices, but He will even help us with the "want-to." It doesn't get any better than this.

God's Word is true, but we often let past guilt or deep feelings of unworthiness rob us of the strength and confidence that connecting with a living God would provide. However, there is hope for our stinkin' thinkin'. First John 3:20 informs us that even when our hearts condemn us, God is greater than our hearts. We can be our own worst enemies. Instead of listening to our own negative self-talk, we can claim the truth of God's Word and recite it until it becomes our new self-talk. It will change the way we live.

## Wounded by the Church

On a regular basis, an anxious, depressed, and wounded person comes into my (Beverly's) office after seeking solace from church folks, only to be toxically shamed and blamed even more. Their encounter left them feeling worse about themselves and God than before they went for help. I heard a saying years ago that "Christians are the only army that kill their wounded." Sadly, that can still be true today.

Maybe you, too, have distanced yourself from the Lord because you have been hurt by the Church or by Christian people. We would like to offer an apology for folks who have failed to represent the love of Jesus to you. They are human and they will let you down, but God never will. Jesus offers up comfort for those who have been hurt or offended by religion or religious practices: "Are you tired? Worn out? Burned out on religion? Come to me. Get away with me and you'll recover your life. I'll show you how to take a real rest. Walk with me and work with me—watch how I do it. Learn the unforced rhythms of grace. I won't lay anything heavy or ill-fitting on you. Keep company with me and you'll learn to live freely and lightly" (Matthew 11:28–30 MSG). Jesus invites those who are disenfranchised with religion or the Church to come to Him.

Whatever misconceptions we have about the Christian walk or a relationship with Him or His people will be answered as we come to "keep company with Him." It is in the quiet moments meditating on Him that we can learn the "unforced rhythms of grace." When we figure out who Christ is and understand the depth of His love and care for us, we aren't afraid to draw close to Him. The benefits we receive from connection with Him can provide confidence in crisis, comfort in the midst of chaos, and peace even in the presence of pain.

## Unanswered Prayer

Perhaps you truly trusted God to answer your prayer and you did not get the answer you wanted. That may have shattered your trust in Him. In our many years of counseling, we have sat across from quite a few folks with fragile faith.

Randy had his dream job working for a large construction company in town. He was let go from his job abruptly, and he never really knew why. His boss told him, "The company decided to go another direction," but that never made sense, since he knew he was doing a great job.

"This isn't fair. My confidence is shot, and I'm so depressed that I don't even feel like going out there to look for another job." Finally, in desperation, he "bit the bullet," as he said and went to work at his brother-in-law's insurance company.

"My pride kept me fighting it for a while because I didn't want to feel like I owed my brother-in-law for giving me a job." To Randy's surprise, he actually liked the business and found out he was really good at it.

In therapy, I (Beverly) helped Randy with perspective. We worked on developing his trust in God's plan, along with unpacking the hurt and bitterness he felt from his untimely job termination.

Six months later, the city of Charlotte was hit with the recession that was sweeping the country. Construction came to a grinding halt, and many companies, including his former one, folded, some even after decades of doing business.

"I'd like to say that they deserve it," Randy reported, "but forgiving them has given me peace. I now see why God allowed me to lose that dream job. I would have never ventured out to try something new, and I would now be in the same sad state as so many people I know who stayed in construction."

## Beverly's Story

I (Beverly) have a story of my own regarding unanswered prayer. It was almost thirty years ago when my husband, Tom, got his second master's degree and was planning on joining me in my counseling practice. In those days we worked from home, and our current house only had one office. So, we started looking for a home with two extra bedrooms that would allow us to work together and be close to our children when they got home from school. There was a builder from Florida who had started building in neighborhoods in North Carolina. We fell in love with a house plan he designed that would be perfect for us. It would create a waiting room and two offices in a finished basement.

Unfortunately, we were quite poor, trying to survive on Tom's pastor salary while we were knee-deep in school debt. We figured that we couldn't afford to live in the ritzy neighborhoods that the Florida builder had chosen in Charlotte. So, we instructed our Realtor to find a good compromise close to the Christian school where our children attended.

Wow, the first week she found one. It had a small basement that needed A LOT of work, but it was doable and the girls could walk to school. *Surely this is God's plan. How could it not be?* we thought. We put in a fair offer and prayed every day and night with the girls and each other that the Lord would give us "our house." We talked about what we would do to fix it up. We discussed how our furniture would fit, what their rooms would look like, and how we would put a play set in the backyard. A few days later, our Realtor called, quite distressed. A fellow Realtor whom she knew had put in a lower bid earlier without telling her, and the seller gave the house to him.

"He bought it right out from under you and me," she said with disbelief. "This is unfair and just plain unethical."
My heart fell into my stomach with disappointment. "You're kidding," was all I could muster. She continued sharing about how she wanted to bring him up on ethics charges with the Board of Realtors. Honestly, she sounded like she was in a barrel as I tuned her out in my own discouraged disillusionment.
*But, Lord, I thought we had this* kept running over and over in my head. *Don't You want us to have a house we can use to minister for You? You can do anything. Why didn't You stop this unethical salesman? Are You even there or for us?*
Memories of all the unanswered prayers I had prayed throughout my lifetime came to mind. (That's just like the sneaky snake, Sa-

tan, isn't it?) I thought about my mother's salvation that was still pending, me not yet getting my PhD, and so many more. Funny, at times like this, we don't look at the list of prayers He does answer, only the ones that make us feel lost and forsaken.

Our sweet godly real estate agent diligently continued to search for us, and five months later she found a house for sale that had been constructed by the builder we loved. We were sure we could not afford it, but it was back in the day when companies bought houses for their executives who needed to relocate. The house was owned by GMAC. It had not been shown in weeks because somehow someone missed the deadline to get it placed in the Multiple Listing Book, the Realtor's Bible before the dawn of the Internet. This was a mistake that the Lord let happen just for us.

On Sunday, we prayed together as a family. Then we put an offer on the house that was extremely low compared to what it was worth. But that was what we could afford. In minutes they took the offer! Not only did we have the ideal home we wanted, in the neighborhood we wanted, but we got it for less than we even thought possible. Only the God of the universe could have created a plan like this for us. The first few years we lived there, we would pull in the driveway and say out loud to each other, "I wonder when the real owners are going to come and kick us out."

We have now been there almost thirty years, and some evenings at dusk, when we have helped a couple get free from toxic thoughts and rebuild trust, or when a person suffering from depression or anxiety walks up the back steps of our basement office, I stop to look at the sunset and thank God that His ways are so much greater than mine.

Often, we can only see right in front of us. We want what we want and get angry with God for not complying with our wishes. But God sees the bigger picture. Isaiah 55 says that God's ways are not our ways and His thoughts are not our thoughts. He knows what's going to happen and He takes care of us, even in spite of ourselves.

## God Has Your Back

No matter what your life situation, remember that you always have an audience with the living God. In Psalm 40:1–3, David, our example writes: "I waited patiently for the LORD; he turned to me and heard my cry. He lifted me out of the slimy pit, out of the mud and mire; he set my feet on a rock and gave me a firm place to stand. He put a new song in my mouth, a hymn of praise to our God" (NIV). Have you ever felt like you're in a slimy pit, that you've been wallowing around in the muck and mire and you can't seem to get your footing? He has guided you to this moment in time to let you know He will lead you out! He will plant your feet on that rock of His salvation and hold you there with His love. No matter where you have been, what you have done or haven't done, the Lord is here for you. Your Divine Daddy's gotcha now, and you're gonna be okay.

Romans 8:38–39 proclaims this truth: "For I am convinced that neither death nor life, neither angels nor demons, neither the present nor the future, nor any powers, neither height nor depth, nor anything else in all creation, will be able to separate us from the love of God that is in Christ Jesus our Lord" (NIV). I think you need to say "amen!" to this out loud right where you are!

Our prayer for you as you establish this empowering relationship with the Creator God is found in Ephesians 3:16–19: "I pray that out of his glorious riches he may strengthen you with power through his Spirit in your inner being, so that Christ may dwell in your hearts through faith. And I pray that you, being rooted and established in love, may have power, together with all God's holy people, to grasp how wide and long and high and deep is the love of Christ, and to know this love that surpasses knowledge—that you may be filled to the measure of all the fullness of God" (NIV).

The Lord is always available, always on the job, but we can fail to notice this unless we are intentional about looking for Him. Needless to say, if our faces are fastened to our phones, if we are constantly compelled to heed the siren call of our digital devices, we can easily miss the most important moments of our lives. We can live

162

our lives either tech-pecked or tuned in to our divine destiny. We pray that this book will help you do the latter.

## Making It Real

1. What is the hardest part about unplugging to plug in to God? Do you find in the moments when you can calm your heart and take time out in the Lord's presence, you are benefited? If so, describe your experience.
2. Do you feel unworthy of God's love? Reread the scriptures listed earlier that define your divine worth.

   - Jeremiah 31:3–4
   - Zephaniah 3:17
   - Zechariah 2:8
   - Deuteronomy 33:27
   - Romans 5:8

Does understanding how God sees you change how you see yourself? Write about that.

3. Do you have you have an unhealthy view of God? If so, where did that view come from? In light of God's Word, what is your opinion now?
4. Do you have difficulty forgiving yourself for past decisions and actions? Reread the scriptures in this chapter about God's thorough forgiveness.

   - 1 John 1:9
   - Psalm 103:1–10, 12
   - Hebrews 8:12

Understanding how fully the Lord forgives you, ask Him to help you write out a prayer to forgive yourself. Live in the light of that forgiveness.

5. Have you ever been hurt by the Church or by people who identify themselves as Christians? Has it kept you from finding fellowship with God's people? Read Hebrews 10:23–25:

"Let us hold fast the confession of our hope without wavering, for He who promised is faithful; and let us consider how to stimulate one another to love and good deeds, not forsaking our own assembling together, as is the habit of some, but encouraging one another; and all the more as you see the day drawing near" (NASB). What does this verse mean to you?

6. Reread Psalm 40:1–3. Claim the victory this verse promises for whatever challenges you are facing in life right now. Claim it for helping you set healthy boundaries with technology. Then you won't live tech-pecked but rather tuned in to God, to the beauty He has created for you, to the real-live face-to-face people He has placed in your life, and with the deeper layers of your own soul.

Thank you for taking this journey with us. Feel our prayers for God to daily bring you His fulfillment and peace as you move from being tech-pecked to being tuned in to Him.

# About the Authors:

Linda Newton and Beverly Rodgers are twin sisters and adult survivors of childhood abuse. As wounded healers, both ladies spend their days leading others to a greater understanding of God's redeeming power. Linda works as a pastoral counselor for a growing church in California and Dr. Beverly runs a thriving counseling practice in Charlotte, North Carolina. Each with thirty plus years in the counseling field, the sisters share with seasoned awareness that there is a bedrock of strength to be found in limiting the draining distractions that prevent cultivating daily intimacy with God.

Beverly is the author of Becoming a Family That Heals, and Linda published 12 Ways to Turn Your Pain Into Praise, both books chronicle each author's journey from heartbreak to healing. While the twins stay connected through digital devices, what they crave most is face-to-face connection, which they make happen by crossing the continent to get together as often as possible.

For additional copies of

# Tech-pecked of Tuned in: Finding God in a Digital World

visit www.amazon.com
(available in printed and Kindle Ebook format)


For more information about Dr. Beverly Rodgers:
visit www.rodgerscc.com

For more information about Linda Newton:
visit www. lindanewtonspeaks.com

# Notes

# Notes

# Notes

# Notes

9 781589 303140